"Alex Mammadyarov is the
she describes the many asp
that is not about passing through anticipated stages but embarking on an open-ended process of personal growth. Written for those still working with an earlier loss, as well as those currently deep in the process, *Growing Through Grief* offers wise companionship that considers all the subtle nuances readers are likely to encounter along the way."

—**Kara Hoppe, MA, MFT**, psychotherapist, death doula, and author of *Baby Bomb*

"*Growing Through Grief* is the book I wish I'd had close by during the quiet, disorienting moments after loss. With tenderness and clarity, Alex Mammadyarov reminds us that grief isn't something we 'get over,' but something we grow through. She holds space for grief's depth and complexity while offering supportive, grounded tools for living inside it. If you're moving through grief or walking beside someone who is, *Growing Through Grief* is a generous guide that offers both comfort and unexpected hope."

—**Cyndie Spiegel**, author of *Microjoys: Finding Hope (Especially) When Life Is Not Okay*

"Alex Mammadyarov is a bright and important new presence in the bereavement field. Her mix of personal experience and professional insight is exactly the kind of combination that will help move the field forward into new arenas. Her book will be a comfort for and an inspiration to every reader."

—**Hope Edelman**, author of *Motherless Daughters: The Legacy of Loss*

"This book is a beautiful and compassionate companion for anyone navigating the terrain of loss. With heartfelt wisdom, clinical insight, and deep humanity, Alex Mammadyarov offers gentle and tender guidance without pressure. A true gift for grievers, this is a validating, supportive, and tenderly honest book. You'll feel seen, not fixed. A necessary balm for aching hearts."

—**Gina Moffa, LCSW**, grief and trauma therapist, and author of *Moving On Doesn't Mean Letting Go*

"Through her own experience of loss, and as a therapist for many grievers, Alex Mammadyarov has written an excellent and practical field guide for the griever who finds themselves in a strange land in which their own reactions—and the reactions of those around them—are surprising, mysterious, and more difficult than they ever imagined."

—**Mary-Frances O'Connor, PhD**, author of *The Grieving Brain* and *The Grieving Body*

"*Growing Through Grief* is a clear-eyed and steady companion for anyone navigating the wilderness of loss. Alex shows us that grief is not a riddle to solve, but a terrain to move through—and, with time, to grow within."

—**Rebecca Soffer**, best-selling author of *The Modern Loss Handbook*

Growing Through Grief

A Compassionate Guide to Finding Meaning and Purpose After Life-Altering Loss

Alex Mammadyarov, LMHC

New Harbinger Publications, Inc.

Publisher's Note

This publication is designed to provide accurate and authoritative information in regard to the subject matter covered. It is sold with the understanding that the publisher is not engaged in rendering psychological, financial, legal, or other professional services. If expert assistance or counseling is needed, the services of a competent professional should be sought.

NEW HARBINGER PUBLICATIONS is a registered trademark of New Harbinger Publications, Inc.

New Harbinger Publications is an employee-owned company.

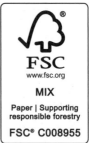

Copyright © 2025 by Alex Mammadyarov
New Harbinger Publications, Inc.
5720 Shattuck Avenue
Oakland, CA 94609
www.newharbinger.com

Cover design by Sara Christian

Acquired by Jennye Garibaldi and Elizabeth Hollis Hansen

Edited by Madison Davis

Library of Congress Cataloging-in-Publication Data on file

FSC
www.fsc.org
MIX
Paper | Supporting responsible forestry
FSC® C008955

Printed in the United States of America

27   26   25

10   9   8   7   6   5   4   3   2   1   First Printing

To Britt and Riyad, whose love and care make this book possible.

For my parents, Karen and Billy Zappala.

CONTENTS

FOREWORD

Grief is a universal experience that completely upends and rearranges our lives. It strips us down and reshapes us in ways we never anticipated. It alters our sense of safety, our understanding of time, and more often than not, our very identity. It is deeply disorienting and overwhelming, and when it comes for you, I want you to reach for this book.

I was initially drawn to Alex and her work on social media. In an age when grifters with big opinions seek to develop (and monetize) catch-all solutions to our complex problems, Alex keeps it real, authentic, and transparent. She does not promise quick fixes but instead commits to walking with you in your grief as you work to discover your own unique path to healing. She is willing to dwell in the complexity of grief—not tidy it up, not push through it for the sake of closure—stay with it, learn from it, and allow it to be a source of connection rather than isolation. That kind of bravery is rare. And that kind of storytelling is necessary.

Her commitment to ensuring that we all have the space we need to grieve, forever, is admirable. This commitment coupled with her actual expertise on grief developed through extensive research, education, and work with private clients made me an instant fan. She is someone who doesn't just get it personally from having lost both of her parents, but she also has the tools, wisdom, and clinical experience to make her a truly trusted source on how to navigate grief and learn to live with loss.

Growing Through Grief is so much more than a self-help book. It is a guide, a roadmap for navigating loss with compassion and grace. Alex and I know from losing our parents that grief lasts forever. It is not easy, and it is not something you get over. Instead, it is something you thoughtfully integrate into your life over and over again, forever. Grief alters how we think, how we feel, how we move through the world, and how we love. Leveraging her clinical and personal experiences this book shows you how to truly live a full life in the midst of devastating loss.

As someone who has spent years writing and speaking about grief, I know how lonely it can feel to live with loss in a culture that so often urges us to "move on." But books like this one push back against that harmful narrative. Instead, they say: Take your time. Feel what you feel. Let your grief be proof of your love.

When you lose someone you love, this book, this gift from Alex, will help you rebuild.

With compassion, grace, and care,

Marisa Renee Lee
Author of *Grief Is Love: Living with Loss*

INTRODUCTION

I don't have a cure for you. Before you shut this book and throw your hands up, I implore you to stick around for a moment and consider this: Grief isn't something to be cured. It is something to grow through. What do I mean by that? With time and practice, the loss you have endured can become woven into your life in such a way that you are not weighed down by suffering. You can remain connected to the person you grieve, never parting with the deep desire for them to be here physically, and yet, you can find a way to continue on. You can tend to the pain so it does not consume all the space inside you—making way for some good and some fulfillment, and (believe it or not) some of the joy that is so vital to life. While I don't have a cure for you, I can offer a perspective that may help you find that a cure is not what you need.

Since you find yourself reading this book, you are probably looking for something and you might not even know what that is, which is okay. I might guess that you are looking for some relief from the weight you feel. Or you have gotten that relief and now wonder what comes next. I also understand that you may not want to get "better." *Better* is loaded. It speaks of time gone by, of accommodating something so wrong that it feels wrong to acclimate to. So, I'm never going to rush you. I'm just going to be here to hold up a mirror, to help you see more clearly what I believe you already know deep inside yourself. I'm just going to offer you invitations along the way, to feel more resourced being with what is, to become curious about the ways that loss has changed you, to connect with some hope. I know how much toxic positivity is lobbed at the grieving, which makes this book a nuanced endeavor. I won't sugarcoat the pain because we need to be honest about it. And hope is important too. Before we go any further, let's back up and create a foundation of shared language.

Finding the Words

Grief is often misunderstood, creating even more confusion about how to cope. Having clarity in the way we talk about it is important. Of course, language is also not a one-size-fits-all tool. By putting words to your experience, you can expand self-knowledge amid all the changes of grief. I encourage you to practice finding the words and trying them on to see which ones feel right. Let's clarify some common terms.

Grief: What It Is and What It Isn't

Grief is not a contained and singular emotional event. It is a vast collection of complex feelings we come to own, always shifting in appearance and shape and depth, forever slipping through the cracks in everything. It is more than just "sadness"—a word sometimes mistakenly used interchangeably.

Grief is universal and unique. Everyone experiences grief at some point in their lives because we all go through at least one life-altering loss. Why? Because it's utterly human to experience connection, love, and attachment—and also utterly human to die. We experience grief in varying magnitudes in various situations in life, however. Living with grief lends an ability to identify less obvious grief where others may not see it. Though this book focuses on grief from death loss, please know that there are many griefs shaped by life. You might think of them as being lowercase "grief" or uppercase "Grief"—and only you can decide which is which.

Grief also does not abide by a timeline. You may have experienced a recent loss or maybe it has been years since it happened. Either way, you are in the right place. You are allowed to start reflecting on and talking about your grief today, even after years of not doing it, even if it comes as a surprise to others. It is never too late to acknowledge that this loss is a significant part of your life. If you are in the earlier days of grief, hearing there is no time limit can make the journey to feeling some semblance of wholeness seem totally unfeasible. Know that grief really does ebb and flow and range in intensity over time, sometimes floating into the background and other times popping up to pay us unexpected visits. It won't always feel like it does right now.

Mourning

Sometimes, grief and mourning are conflated with each other. Let's make a distinction here. *Mourning* is the outward expression of sorrow for a loved one who has died. It is a word associated with the conventions and practices that display our grief, which is the multitude of feelings we hold on the inside. Notice an image coming to mind. Maybe people wearing black at a funeral, which is where we receive the most attentiveness from others. But that attentiveness tends to drop off as we continue to grieve though not outwardly mourn.

Talking About Their Death

There is no right or wrong way to verbalize how your loved one came to no longer be here. The most common ways we hear this expressed are "He died" or "They passed away." In this book, I will more often say "died." When I was younger, a rebellious part of me took offense to "passing away," as it sounded so gentle compared to how final and unforgiving loss can feel. There is something somewhat softer about "passing," which may be the language that feels most comfortable for you. This is okay too, so long as it is not language you are adopting for the comfort of others. More on this later.

Another word you may notice often is "lost." To be clear, this is meant to represent that you have lost the ability to be in physical proximity with them. This does not mean that their essence, your connection with them, is ever, ever lost—on the contrary. More on this later too.

Meaning and Purpose

Meaning is not something we are required to find after loss, but many people do end up looking for it. It usually begins with the ever unanswered, perpetually frustrating question: *Why?* Meaning-making may seem designed to answer this question but, really, we never get the answer and—for the record—it shouldn't have happened. Meaning-making is about deciding what the loss means for us and our lives going forward.

Creating purpose after loss answers the question, *What am I going to do now?* The loss doesn't serve a purpose—we do. When my mother was dying, my sister asked her, "How am I going to do this? How am I going to live without you?" She was only twenty-five years old and preparing to be my legal guardian. My mother told her that I would give her purpose. My mother wasn't telling my sister that becoming my guardian was the *reason* she was dying, that it was some grand lesson concocted by her illness. Caring for me was simply what my sister was going to do with this loss.

We're going to sift through the changes together to help you build more self-awareness and self-compassion. Finding meaning and purpose isn't all about discovery—it's also something we create. You are by no means required to turn your pain into purpose or to grow through it. But opening yourself to this possibility may help you feel that life, with all its grief, is still worth it. Mostly, grief creates a lot of change without our say-so. It changes just about everything, stripping down all the layers and bringing us right to our core. I'd like to empower you to regain some of your agency.

How to Use This Book

To bring some of the major themes of loss and grief to life, I will be drawing from my own experience, as well as the clinical experience I have sought out and continue to pursue. From time to time, you will read some case stories. These are composites built from my work companioning the grieving over several years and none represent any single, specific person. Throughout this book, I will share suggestions for coping. Think of these suggestions as offerings. I do not mean to create work for you as you grieve. If the offerings don't apply, let them pass over you. If they don't fit for the moment but intrigue you, take note of them for later and trust they will come back to you if needed. If you don't need a suggestion and feel supported enough by seeing your experience reflected on the page, then we have done something meaningful here—me writing to you and you reading. Please note that there are also free tools that accompany this book and are available online at http://www.newharbinger.com/55787. Wherever you are with your grief, let's be present right here in the beginning, as we turn to it together now.

CHAPTER 1

The New Normal

Here you are at the crossroads. The worst thing that could happen has happened. Someone in your life, totally irreplaceable, who you've only ever known to be living and breathing here beside you, has died. It is the unimaginable, the event others respond to by saying "I can't imagine it," although you wish they would try instead of saying that. You never could imagine it either—now you are here in the thick, heavy realness of it. If initially people showed up for you, perhaps that support has faded in the unspoken and guaranteed way that it does. Maybe you have tried to go back to whatever "normal" is and do what is expected of you. It may feel like something is off, beyond missing your person, as though this way of continuing forward is not working. Maybe you're not even sure what "working" means. It may feel like something is lurking below the surface, probably a whole lot of grief. I have been at this crossroads myself, where the tectonic plates beneath my life started to shift and whether or not I was ready, I had to move with them.

It is the night before my college graduation. After having dinner with my family, who are in town for the festivities, I return to my boyfriend's apartment. I find myself sitting alone in his room, on the edge of the bed. As the sun sets over the Hudson River, I am struck by a mixture of deep sadness and dread that I can't fully grasp or name. It's gnawing at my stomach and tightening in my throat and stinging my eyes. *They're really not coming back.*

This is the thought I take away from this night, this weekend, and if I'm being honest, this celebration. It's not as though I'm entrenched in the magical thinking after loss that Joan Didion describes. I've had years to commit to memory and understanding that my parents really are dead. However, something about the eve of a milestone, a major accomplishment—one they would and should be here to celebrate but cannot—just does not ring true. It's as though in some deeper layer of my mind and soul, I was anticipating their arrival at the ceremony.

I make some semblance of peace with this. I try to appreciate the celebration and lean into the presence of the family members who are able to physically partake. These efforts don't fully ameliorate the sadness that hangs out in the background like an uninvited guest, but they do help somewhat. Unbeknownst to me, I am not just graduating from college, but from a phase of running away from my grief.

When I was fifteen, I went back to school two weeks after my mother died following a five-year struggle with breast cancer, which began just a year after my father died from esophageal cancer. Over the next four years, I grappled with the following: On one hand, I had this sense that none of the silly maladies of the teen years really mattered. On the other, I really *was* my chronological age and wanted to be like everyone else. With weekly therapy sessions and family support, I trudged through an attempt at normalcy and pretty successfully pulled it off. Toward the end, college admissions provided a ticket outside my hometown bubble and also a breath of relief. I believed that I was known for these sad things that had happened to me, maybe even pitied. New York City provided a chance to share my story on my own terms, I thought, or to run away from it entirely. Moving was an opportunity to distance myself from my grief...until it came roaring back as I sat on the edge of that bed. Something had clearly shifted, and it felt worth investigating.

A few months after graduation, I went to a retreat for women who lost their mothers in childhood. I was shy, a little wide-eyed, and at times totally flooded with emotion. My voice caught in my throat when I tried to speak. I was also the youngest one there. One afternoon, someone took me aside and told me, "You're probably thinking, *Oh no, I'm still going to be grieving when I'm fifty.*" I heard that yes, probably I would still be grieving, and yes, that would be okay. The women in that group were doing themselves a service I would come to revere. They recognized that it did not matter how many years had gone by since they lost their mothers. They had grown through a grief that was ongoing and worthy of continued processing.

So is yours. However, dominant culture makes little room for true grief processing and instead encourages us to "move on." These are two words that ring so hollow when it comes to parting with a person we deeply love. When someone dies, we are usually given the bulk of the support we are going to get in the very beginning. Then it drops off fairly soon as people resume their lives. When you are the one living with the loss, there is no resume button. This is now life, and it can feel absolutely terrifying. One way we can make sense of this reaction to loss is to view it in the context of a society that truly fears vulnerability.

There are culturally diverse responses to death and loss worldwide, and North American society doesn't let us grieve for decades or a lifetime, just perhaps a few weeks or months. When we are in grief, we are at our most raw. As much as the tide continues to thankfully turn, and mental health conversations take center stage, we still have decades upon decades of unlearning to do. The pressure to white-knuckle our way through grief is there because we struggle to witness one another in our vulnerability. It is so hard to be with what cannot be fixed when, in the digital age, we have access to solutions at our fingertips all the time. It is easier to avert our eyes and hope people figure out how to deal with it, or hide it away so we can stop experiencing the discomfort that arises when we don't feel useful to others.

Regardless of whether your loss occurred months or years ago, you may have attempted to return to "normal," perhaps feeling the pressure of this grief-phobic society. Or maybe because you are yearning for some relief. It is an understandable wish. *Maybe if I try to act normally, it will all be okay.* Like pushing against a current, these efforts may have revealed the ways in which grief sticks around, strikes back intensely, or more stealthily creeps up on you even as you try to bury it.

What Happens When We Avoid Grief

You might think that turning away from your grief will allow it to fade. Though you might wish this to be true, the reality is that the grief will continue to live inside you, burrowed in your subconscious, stored in your body. Until you honor its existence and develop the skill of sitting with it, a number of challenges may arise. Here are some of those effects.

When the grief takes the color away: Since the loss, you may have found yourself just going through the motions, as the vibrancy of life leaves your world. On the outside, it may seem as though you are coping, but your inner experience is foggy. A sense of emptiness spreads out into everything.

When the grief breaks through: You may have had to return to work before you feel ready and as a result, find yourself flooded in the break-room or the bathroom. The same may happen at social gatherings or anywhere out in the world, when least expected.

When the grief pushes you away from others: Unprocessed grief has a tremendous effect on our interior selves and thus, our relation-ships. You may feel isolated from friends and have difficulty under-standing how to show up in new or existing relationships while feeling like a different person.

When the grief makes you question it all: You may have recently asked yourself, *What's the point?* You might feel this about work, your plans, life itself. You may question your faith or spirituality, even feeling betrayed by your beliefs. Too much time spent feeling disconnected from the point of our lives can lead us into darker and more detrimental places.

When the grief hides like a ticking time bomb: It's common to throw yourself into distraction overdrive through work, reaching for each monkey bar of achievement until, eventually, there is a fall. We also avoid through caretaking and many will numb through alcohol and other substances.

None of these actions, findings, or sensations are markers of failure. These are natural responses you may feel to loss. You might be thinking: *Of course there's no color in my world. She* was *the color in my world.* Of course, grief overwhelms our bodies and makes it scary to be vulnerable with others. It raises innumerable questions and creates a temptation to distract from the most delicate wound. There's more here than the fact that grief is too much to avoid; it is so worthy of being tended to. Grief will show up one day, whether you turn toward it or not. In all likelihood, it is probably already here, manifesting in ways that only the little voice inside you can recognize. What to do with it all can feel daunting. Being here, right now, reading these pages, is you taking your first step.

Grief and Expectations

A common phrase among early grief initiates is, *I just wish there was some sort of guide for this.* The death of a loved one can leave us so wildly untethered. When a client shares this wish with me, I sometimes wish I could offer more than validation. Though grievers can be helped, grief is not something to be fixed. Sometimes people turn to models of grief to try to understand where they are, what might come next, and grasp at some control. Today, the most-known model of grief

is the Five Stages: denial, anger, bargaining, depression, and acceptance. Created by Swiss-American psychiatrist and innovator of death
studies, Elisabeth Kübler-Ross, it was first published in her 1969 book
On Death and Dying. Reading through those five words, you have
probably thought or said something to the effect of:

I don't know what stage I'm in.

I was feeling depressed but now I'm angry again.

I don't think I could ever accept that they're gone.

What does bargaining even mean?

The Five Stages, as they are used today, often lead to confusion for
grieving people who notice that the stages happen out of order or even
become cyclical. It might feel confining to imagine that there is a step-
by-step progression of bereavement, and therefore a "right" and
"wrong" way to grieve. The last thing that we need to feel when we are
already in the depths of sorrow is self-criticism for being there.
Elisabeth Kübler-Ross didn't create this model to restrict grieving
people——she actually didn't create it to describe bereavement at all. It
was actually derived from her work with the dying, as they processed
and tried to make peace with their own impending deaths. So, if you
have struggled to find where you fit among the stages, this would make
sense. If you relate to parts of it, then it may be a wonderful source of
grounding and awareness. You can say to yourself, for instance, *Okay,
I am back in the anger.* The key is to remember that grief is fluid and
because we continue on living, old stages will probably resurface.

Newer research has tried to make sense of the way we grieve.
Psychologist J. William Worden (2009) created the Four Tasks of
Mourning. The tasks are as follows:

Task 1: Accept the reality of the loss

Task 2: Process the pain of the loss

Task 3: Adjust to a world without the deceased

Task 4: Find an enduring connection with the deceased in the midst of embarking on a new life

Worden takes care to emphasize that these tasks can be returned to and completed more than once throughout your life. Even in its final task, the model does not feel finite, as though grief is a closed book.

Further back, in 1999, psychologists Dr. Margaret Stroebe and Dr. Henk Schut published the Dual Processing Model of Bereavement. Stroebe and Schut sought to provide a clear explanation for how people actually process grief. They found that life after loss consists of two types of stressors: loss-oriented and restoration-oriented. People regulate themselves by oscillating between the two (Stroebe and Schut 1999). This means people sometimes avoid and, at other times, confront their grief head-on, experiencing doses of it in order to keep going. Unfortunately, these models tend to remain most known within clinical and academic circles, rarely making it into the mainstream. They affirm the idea of a new normal that so many need to hear is okay. I'm here to tell you this: It is okay.

Reframing the Road Ahead

Maybe this loss isn't what you thought it would be or maybe you didn't think about what it would be like at all. Most of us don't truly consider what it would be like to experience world-shattering grief, until it actually happens inside our own life. Grief is something for other people, out there, until we ourselves become the *other people*. Maybe when the loss first occurred, you were quick to look toward the future, where this pain is not so sharp and searing. Maybe you were focusing on putting one foot in front of the other each day and the thought of the future, unclear without them, raised fear. However you have been approaching your path so far, I am going to give you some words of permission so that we can reframe the road ahead.

How am I going to move past this?

You're not. You're going to move with it. This is a time to start approaching your own emotions with openness and curiosity, even if it feels scary, even if you can only do it in those little doses. Together, we are going to continue checking in with your grief, asking about what it needs, and considering how you can give it what it needs—all in order to keep yourself free from more suffering.

How am I going to go back to who I was before this?

You're not. You are probably never going to return to the person you were prior to the loss. Something is unequivocally different now and likely, so are you. Your concept of grief may have to expand, as you are not only grieving the person you lost but also who you were. You will not just be losing, though. As you let parts of the former you go, you will start to meet an emerging version of yourself. It may just be difficult to see the new you right now.

The idea that you are not going to return to "normal" may be a hard pill to swallow. You might notice some resistance to this idea because it's scary to consider that you could experience any further loss than you have already. The degree to which people change after loss varies, let's be totally clear, so this isn't to say that you are an entirely new human. You may just gain some new parts and feel disconnected from others. Let's step back to consider why this might be, and look at how your life may have been changed by loss. Whether the loss of a parent, a child, partner, sibling, other family member, or friend, it's likely that you will identify with more than one of the secondary losses—something you lost because of the Big Loss. You may have lost:

- A sense of belonging or safety

- Shared memories

- Potential for vital conversations

- Parts of identity or culture

- Connections to meaningful places

- Family lore, recipes, or medical history

- Their witnessing of future milestones

- Their unique love and support

- Answers to your questions

- Shared future experiences

- Guidance in phases of development

- Opportunities for shared healing

Notice the secondary losses that resonate for you. If you feel called, take note of them in your journal. If this leads you into a larger free-write journal entry, allow it. Get curious and see what comes up. Or just writing the bullet points may be enough for right now.

After all this loss, it's normal to reflect on who you have been and question who are you are going to be now. So much of our sense of who we are is tied to other people. Even the most introverted of us are, in some way, social creatures with identities that are in part informed by our relationships. When a loved one who may have provided a connection to family history and culture dies, it can feel as though you are standing at one end of a collapsed bridge. You are tasked with the arduous job of rebuilding it, if and when you want to. When a loved one is not here to answer your questions and provide guidance, you are left to sort through the process of finding yourself without a home base to remind you who you have always been. You may feel stark *before* and *after* identities around loss. For me, loss was a formative factor in my development, something I grew up *with*. So I could better understand, put words to, and navigate it over time and with intentional practice. Perhaps because of my decades-long experiment, I believe we all have the capacity to grow with our grief.

As you consider the list of secondary losses, it may feel painful to see the larger scope of what your loss has entailed on paper. I draw your attention here, not to make you feel worse, but to validate what I imagine you are already experiencing. The idea that we can just return to business as usual after losing someone almost becomes silly when we take what that loss really means and lay it out on the table. Grief stretches over the expanse of our lives and seeps into the little cracks inside everything. There is no going back to normal. An entirely new normal (if we can even call it that) has formed. We need another way of dealing with grief, a deeper way, one that gets down into the roots, helps us stretch up into the sky, and breathe again.

Growing Through Grief

The phrase *growing through grief* means healing through loss by making an intentional choice to not push it away and to instead embrace the truth that life is now entirely different, as are we. It is a brave act of surrender, waving a white flag in the face of every temptation to suppress your emotions. It may not feel like it right now, but by choosing the way of integration, you are really just choosing yourself. You are choosing you in the same way the elder women in my grief retreat group chose themselves at fifty and their inner, younger selves forty and thirty and twenty and ten. I imagine their child selves awestruck by a room full of people sharing the same pain, one maybe seldom discussed in some of their homes. I also imagine a version of you, decades from now, remembering yourself in this moment and feeling grateful that you chose to follow the voice inside saying *there has to be a different way.*

Integrating grief is not only about embracing the truth that we have been changed by loss. We also choose growth because we acknowledge that grief lasts for the rest of our lives. Our grief is ongoing, though shapeshifting, because our loss is ongoing. We do not grieve and then stop grieving because we do not lose someone and then stop experiencing the loss of them. We may have to do most of the heavy lifting in our grief work in the beginning, but it is a practice that carries us throughout a life with loss. This work is a balancing act at a very precious intersection. It's where we honor our deep disappointment, our sadness, and our rage, and also lean into the belief that good things, things other than pain and loss, are still possible for us. This is how we move forward—a place I know you may not want to go.

When working with someone who is in grief, one of my primary goals is to meet them where they are. This is essential because all people do not want the same things from grief therapy. If I were to divide it very broadly, some people want to move toward relief, maybe even with a sense of urgency. Others just want validation for being exactly where they are, not necessarily ready to feel better. Before we go anywhere, stop to notice what might be coming up for you. If any particular words in the last paragraph stand out, write them in a journal, as well as any feelings they stir up. All you have to do for now is observe.

Relief, Frustration, and Fear

There are probably a whole host of feelings you might have in response to this idea of integrating your grief and growing through it. There might be a sense of relief. No, you do not have to move on and pretend that everything is back to normal. Yes, everything you are feeling makes sense. Grief is not pathology nor a sign of dysfunction. It is exactly what is supposed to happen, although of course you wish it wouldn't, when someone you deeply love dies. It's actually a vital, although painful, process of being fully human. It is a temperature check, although a cruel one, on your ability to feel. It is just evidence that your mind is comprehending devastating loss, that your soul has felt aligned with another, and that your heart is beating. It is devastating, I know, and the relieving part is that you don't have to ignore it.

You might feel frustration. When we lose someone and realize just how painful loss actually is, we feel justifiably angry. It can feel like such an unfair card to be dealt. On top of that, you are breaking through this myth that things go back to normal afterward. What you are embarking upon is quiet work that largely goes unseen. Once you acknowledge that grief is something to be embraced, you will gain a superpower for seeing all the places and spaces and ways it is overlooked. Ultimately, you might also feel frustrated by the idea of even having to continue feeling grief.

The beginnings of integrating grief can also bring up a lot of fear. The "forever of it all" is scary. I felt it when I realized my dead parents weren't coming to my college graduation, and I felt it when I stepped into the room at the grief retreat. The idea that grief lasts as long as loss does can be validating and it can also ring an alarm bell of dread. It doesn't have to. The grief lasts, yes, but it also changes shape as we grow and change with it. Although it will stay with you, it will not always feel the exact way that it does right now.

Using Radical Acceptance

So, what do we do with all these feelings? What I encourage you *not* to do is judge them. Allow them to come up as they do, witness them, and watch them fall away. Notice how one feeling doesn't remain completely permanent in every moment. Part of living a healthy coexistence with grief is practicing radical acceptance of it. *Radical acceptance* is a term coined by Dr. Marsha Linehan, the creator of dialectical behavioral therapy (DBT). Many grieving people struggle with the word "accept" as it arises in conversations around loss. It can carry this connotation that we are somehow saying it is okay that a person has died. Dr. Linehan (2015) makes a point to state that to *accept* something does not mean to *approve* of it but to *align* ourselves with reality in order to reduce our suffering. When we accept that our grief is here to stay, in some capacity, we are being with what is so that we can heal instead of denying the truth with fingers crossed that it goes away. Accepting the presence of our grief also means accepting the presence of all these other feelings that come up along the way. Radical acceptance may also be helpful if any of the models of grief mentioned earlier in this chapter seem aligned, but that word "acceptance" doesn't sit right with you.

Final Thoughts

Where do we go from here? Now that you have acknowledged that you don't have to push the grief down and push yourself through, you can begin practicing some radical acceptance of where you are. No longer at the crossroads, you are here in the new normal. Throughout the remainder of the book, we will explore what happens in the immediate aftermath of loss, the ensuing survival mode, and how to navigate what feels totally unnavigable. We will consider how to self-advocate as you return to work and your social world, and how to ride the waves of grief and changes to your relationships. Toward the end of the book, we will find ways that you can maintain a connection to the person you lost, process and make space for all the ways you have changed, and maybe even support others who grieve. Take it at your own pace. Growing through grief is sacred work and it is the healing work of a lifetime. But today is as good a day as any to begin.

REFLECTION QUESTION

Think back to what you were told about grief before ever living through it yourself. Now that you have experienced it, how many myths about grief can you spot?

CHAPTER 2

The Loss and the Aftermath

I'm eight years old in my parent's bedroom, sometime between April and the cusp of summer. My mother and I are making the bed, lifting and floating the soft, cream-colored sheets.

I ask her, "Is he going to die?" I can see her looking tenderly at me. "Yes," she says.

It's a foggy memory for me. How much was I able to take in, about what this meant? How did I even know to ask the question? Was it part of a larger conversation we were having? Did I prompt her out of the blue? What was I observing through changes to our household dynamic as he declined? I cannot recall like my sister can. She was about to turn twenty and was abroad at the time. They phoned and told her about our dad's illness, saying "You need to come home."

I reach back in my mind for fragments: Peering out one of the front windows, mesmerized by the way the red and blue lights of the ambulance shined on the brick pathway from our door to the street. Feeling hesitation to hug him before leaving for day camp—despite having been his shadow all my life—as he smiled with eyes slightly glazed over, maybe after his stroke. Some of the contextual details from this time will be forever hazy but the feelings, the sensations—those parts remain with clarity. Before long, my mother is calling me out of the pool on a balmy July evening as the sun hangs low and the sky starts to darken. Wrapped in a towel, I sit on her lap, and through some exchange of words I'll never recall, she communicates that my father has died. Everything changes.

Where to Begin

The day someone we love dies it feels like we are born all over again. It's like we must learn how to navigate the world, and really our existence, for the first time. A multitude of ebbing and flowing emotions may feel overwhelming or even unfamiliar as they take up residence inside us. There are new or amplified relational dynamics unfolding, and even our brains struggle to register our surroundings. In this chapter, I will describe some of the emotions and experiences commonly felt and encountered in my clinical practice. Whether you are moving through a loss that has recently occurred or you too are looking back through memory fragments, my wish is that you will find validation and greater clarity about your experience from these pages. We will take it piece by piece.

Different losses create different experiences. Some emotions are often associated with deaths that are anticipated, and other emotions are often associated with deaths that are unexpected. Of course, there is significant overlap here. For instance, *trauma*—emotional distress that overwhelms any built-in capabilities we have to cope—can arise from both sudden and anticipated losses. We often hear "trauma" and think of a singular event, however, the helplessness of witnessing the slow deterioration of a loved one could also overload the ability to cope. As you read, you may notice yourself taking a mental inventory of what does and does not resonate. It is valuable for you to have this information about your own experience. However, I encourage you to check in about any self-judgments that may begin to arise as you take stock. There is no right or wrong way to feel or experience loss.

Anticipatory Grief

When someone comes to me for grief support after experiencing an anticipated loss, they often express that they have already been grieving. We can think of anticipatory grief like a slow drip of grief that becomes accelerated upon the actual passing, amassing into a flood that fills the room. Or we can think of anticipatory grief like Grief: The Prologue or Grief: Act I. It contains some facets of bereavement, yet not others that will be felt once living in the reality of their absence.

Losing Them Before We Lose Them

How is it that we can grieve before a loss has actually happened? Well, we may lose parts of them while they are still here, in the process of leaving. Few people, if anyone, understand this more than those who love and care for someone with Alzheimer's disease, a progressive form of dementia that affects memory, thinking, and behavior. An entire chapter alone could be devoted to the very specific pain of witnessing this confusion and becoming lost along with their person's ability to remember.

We may also lose shared activities. The person you are grieving may not have been able to engage in pastimes you once bonded over. These could be as strenuous as hiking and as simple as talking over coffee at the kitchen table. We may also lose parts of our overall relationship dynamic with them. For instance, as an adult child, there may be a role reversal in which you become the parent to your parent. They may have less capacity to act in the ways that you have always known them to act. The illness and then the impending loss often takes center stage, shifting all the everyday variables. There is certainly loss before the ultimate loss.

Trying to Prepare

Like bracing for impact, we may find ourselves trying to prepare for ultimate loss. Days before my mother's death, I fervently tried to imagine how I would feel afterward. I didn't only imagine it, I tried to actually bring myself into the feeling. I remember wanting to harness all the pain and step inside it while she was still alive, so that she could hold and soothe me through it. It was a creative way of attempting to cope ahead. My thinking was that if I could capture the feeling of being in the pain while she held me, I could feel that hold later while I was alone. Sometimes I hear this early in grief work with clients, either before the loss or shortly thereafter—a desire get ahead of the sorrow that awaits as the reality continues to sink in. The calculus seems to be, *If I know what lies ahead, I can expect it, and maybe even lessen the blow of those feelings.* When I let my mother hold me those days before her death, I was certainly feeling grief—I knew what it meant to be without a parent—but unfortunately, I couldn't truly know how it would feel to be without *her* until I lived it.

On Alert

What underlies this determined preparation is an awareness that our time with a loved one is coming to a close. This is one of the uniquely painful, perhaps even unbearable, parts of anticipated loss. In the week leading up to my mother's death, I struggled with a state of hyper-alert consciousness. There was no leaving her room without saying "I love you," because it could always be the last time we would exchange those words. There was no watching a movie because then I couldn't watch her breathing before I would forget what this looked like. There was no closing my eyes because then she would disappear. Without any guarantee of when it would happen, we neared the place where there is no "later." This awareness can even trigger *fight-flight-freeze* responses, our body's automatic responses to a perceived threat—in this case, the threat is impending loss. The tortuous waiting game of anticipation and the heightened mind-body response to it is very taxing.

FIGHT-FLIGHT-FREEZE

We have remnants of our ancestor's survival strategies. Our sympathetic nervous system becomes activated in response to danger, in order to fight, flee, or freeze when neither fight nor flee is an option. Here's what happens inside the body:

- Cortisol, our stress hormone, and adrenaline are released
- Our heart rate and breathing speed up
- Our pupils dilate
- Our mouths become dry
- Our muscles become tense

Here's what to do about it:

When we are in a fight-flight-freeze state, we are not grounded in our bodies. We may feel anxious, out of control, or dissociated. The most important thing we can do is safely feel back into the present moment, inside our bodies, with a grounding exercise. Here is the 5-4-3-2-1 technique, created by psychotherapist Betty Alice Erickson, for you to try the next time you find yourself activated. Identify the following:

- What are 5 things you can see?
- What are 4 things you can touch?
- What are 3 things you can hear?
- What are 2 things you can smell?
- What is 1 thing you can taste?

Meeting Relief

At some point, our preparation is brought to an end. I struggled to brace against the future pain until the night my sister appeared by my bed and told me, "She's gone." I fell into a deep sleep, finally relieved of my duty, giving up watch because it was now unnecessary. When they eventually leave us, the worst has happened, yet we are able to stop the exhausting work of preparing. This is relief. Relief is one of the more challenging emotions to voice, as it is often accompanied by a secondary feeling of shame. *How could I be relieved by their death?* This is a notion to reframe. We are not relieved by the loss itself but certainly by the loss of the acute stress we were under while waiting for it. When reflecting on the relief, it is important to summon self-compassion. You can do so by imagining how you would respond to a cherished friend in your shoes or by calling in the voice of your loved one. Would you feel judgment toward your friend for their relief or would you maybe even feel relief *for* them? When you get quiet and imagine the voice of your loved one, do you hear them feeling betrayed or might they even understand your relief? You may also not experience relief. Instead, hypervigilance may continue, giving way to a fear of other loved ones dying. This is something we'll explore more as we discuss relationship changes.

Sudden Loss

For many, a loss is entirely unanticipated and we are unprepared. There are various forms of unexpected death, including those due to suicide, a sudden health event or previously undetected illness, pregnancy loss, an accident, homicide, or natural disaster. Just as anticipatory grief contains its own set of intricacies, so too does sudden grief.

A Shock to the Systems

When it comes to sudden loss, there is no plan. This is what makes grief stemming from such a loss uniquely harrowing. There is, generally, no Grief: The Prologue or Grief: Act I. When we discover that someone has died suddenly, we are stripped of any opportunity to process that grief was on its way to us. This discovery can take several forms: receiving the news, happening upon the scene, or being present when it happens. All three push the door wide open for sympathetic nervous system activation. Your heartrate may increase as your thoughts race, your breathing becoming shallow. You may experience tunnel vision and someone may remark that you look pale. These are just some of the physiological reactions that occur when the body registers this threatening event. In this state of overwhelm, we might feel numb. To have life shift so suddenly and to lack information can create a deep sense of everything being surreal and out of control.

Without having any sense of a plan, this may mean having a less prepared support system. Although only so much emotional preparation can be done, there is a scaffolding that family and community can provide when we know loss is impending. With anticipated deaths, sometimes, though not always, loved ones come together to bolster support for those closest to the dying. With sudden loss, instead there may be scrambling to unite as time ticks and calls for arrangements press amidst this still unthinkable loss. There may even be a lack of unification entirely. Those most impacted by the loss suffer without a safety net.

Post-Traumatic Stress

Whether you learn of the death from someone else, are present as it suddenly occurs, or happen upon the scene, all three heart-rending scenarios also make way for trauma. It is greatly distressing to be present during traumatic events or to learn that they have happened to a close family member or friend. Some who experience sudden loss will encounter grief complicated by post-traumatic stress disorder (PTSD). People diagnosed with PTSD present with various symptoms for over one month that are directly connected to a traumatic event and cause clinically significant distress (APA 2013). These symptoms fall into four categories:

- **Intrusive** symptoms can include distressing memories or dreams. Do you experience flashbacks that bring you back as if you are experiencing the news all over again?

- **Avoidant** symptoms include avoiding stimuli (people, places, things) that remind us of the event. Have you been staying away from a place you need to visit, like a doctor's office, because it feels tied to the loss?

- **Negative changes to thoughts and mood**, perhaps feeling detached from others. Think about recent instances of being with your people. Have you found it challenging to feel any sense of connection to them?

- **Arousal,** such as an exaggerated startle response. Have you noticed yourself jumping at the sound of something familiar, like an alarm clock?

In order for a person to receive a PTSD diagnosis, a certain number of symptoms must be present in each category. These questions are not meant to be a diagnostic tool. They offer topics for reflection and discussion with a mental health professional.

Traumatic loss creates an added long-term processing layer for grievers. In the immediate sense, trauma can block painful feelings and memories. But while protective, that can hinder integrating the loss over time. It becomes necessary to work on allowing these memories to surface enough to become somewhat less charged and somewhat more tolerable to be with (Shulman 2018). To be clear, not all who experience sudden loss develop PTSD and what is traumatic for one person may not be for another. Perceptions of an event and abilities to cope vary from person to person. This book alone is not a sufficient resource for managing PTSD. You would be better supported by a combination of trauma-focused therapy and somatic practices.

Feeling Robbed: No Time for a "Good Death"

When a sudden loss occurs, it often contains other losses within it, like the opportunity for your loved one to have a "good death." It might feel understandably strange to read those two words next to each other. According to the Institute of Medicine, "[A] *decent or good* death is one that is: free from avoidable distress and suffering for patients, families, and caregivers; in general accord with patients' and families' wishes; and reasonably consistent with clinical, cultural, and ethical standards" (Emanuel and Emanuel 1998). I first heard this phrase from death doula and attorney Alua Arthur. It's important to acknowledge that not all are afforded their preference of death circumstances due to suddenness or systemic racism and other forms of oppression that affect the care individuals receive. A good death is also subjective, given our varying cultures, values, and beliefs. With sudden loss, there is little, if any, time or space for this. Outside of any comfort we might find in knowing there was not prolonged suffering, it is hard to argue that a sudden death could ever be "good." If your loss was anticipated or even unfolded peacefully, you still may not see it as having been a "good death." That is more than okay.

Many people who grieve sudden losses feel justifiably robbed of their goodbye. It is devastating to acknowledge there being no parting words, no last questions or advice touchstones, no embrace during which both parties know it is the final one. If you are reading this as you grieve a loss that was unanticipated, know that your pain is seen. This is a distinctive anguish so worthy of being held.

If it has been a long time since your loss, how does it feel to read some of your experience reflected here? If your loss was expected, consider how this anticipation shaped your daily life and whether its effects are lingering. If your loss was sudden and you are struggling with shock or fight-or-flight responses, it may be helpful to begin focusing more on the connection between your mind and body.

Grief: A Collection of Emotions

Grief is our internal experience of loss, and it contains a multitude of emotions, so this section is by no means exhaustive. In the beginning, you may actually experience an absence of any emotions at all. As you read on about the emotional experience of initial grief, notice how it feels to be in your body.

Absence of Emotion

You may not be feeling much of anything at all in the aftermath of your loss. If you knew the loss was coming, you may have experienced a build-up of anticipation about what you might feel, only to find that this did not hold true on the other side. Noticing an absence of the sadness or anger you anticipated might begin to stir some self-judgment. I invite you to consider that you have never before been without your loved one in this way. It is too vast to comprehend in the beginning. This natural buffer from the raw emotion may even be protective right now.

Regret

Regret is one of the thornier emotions that can arise both before and after loss, particularly when grappling with choice. When someone in our world is dying, the stakes and what we do with them feel higher than ever. *Do I become the caretaker? Do I opt to not get involved? Do I make amends or maintain my boundaries?* When people ask themselves these questions regarding their choices, they are trying to understand what they feel is their responsibility and they are also trying to mitigate the potential for regret. The challenge here is twofold: We cannot entirely predict our feelings. And with every choice taken or not taken, there may *still* be some regret. For instance, choosing to not say goodbye before a passing may lead to guilt and then regret, though choosing to do so may lead to the formation of trauma and then regret. We can only do what we can with the information and instincts we have in the moment, remembering this compassionately in retrospect.

Guilt

So often regret's companion is guilt. Though everyone who encounters loss can and may experience it, this particular emotion is often expressed by those who have lost a loved one after a battle with mental health challenges and addiction. It may surface as survivor's guilt for some grievers who were present when the loss occurred. Other grievers may feel an overwhelming wish to have been there to somehow prevent it from happening. Feeling a sense of responsibility after loss may also be connected to childhood and your role within your family of origin, perhaps being the eldest or acting as such, tending to everyone else's needs. Grief guilt can manifest as mentally replaying events and asking questions that sound like: *What could I have done differently? Could I have done more?* It may also arise as an imbalanced focus on your perceived shortcomings in your relationship with the loved one you lost.

Anger

The early emotional stirrings of grief are not all melancholic. The death of someone so integral to your world just feels wrong. This can spark a deep sense of injustice. When it dawns upon us that loss isn't reversible, that there is no way to get them back, that we have all these feelings inside that there is no familiar solution for, we may even feel rage. Sometimes, anger is a shield for sadness—particularly if sadness was not acceptable to express growing up. Sometimes, however, anger is just anger. We don't have to diminish its presence or call it something else. This is an emotion that you may not feel immediately but notice later when the loss begins to sink further into the details of your daily life. It may simmer below the surface, flaring when it feels as though others simply do not understand.

Longing

Ultimately, we just want our loved one. It is as simple and as searing as that. We long to be with them, wherever we believe they may be, and we long to have them still here in our world. I regret (only because of how overwhelming this may be) to inform you that in truth, we never stop wanting them. I do not regret to inform you, however, that this is okay. As time moves and we long for them in new and sustained ways, we also adapt to that sensation of longing. This is a testament to a connection that never ends.

Check in with yourself, before we move any further. Take a moment to sit with the various emotions and contemplate your own experience. Which feeling is most salient for you?

Encountering the Aftermath

In the aftermath of the loss, you may notice the first clues that grief is a multifaceted experience. Emotionally, cognitively, and relationally, there are new dynamics taking shape in the minutes, hours, and days that follow a loss.

Emotionally: Fear of "Taking the Lid Off"

When you checked in with yourself about how it felt to read through the various emotions that may arise in the wake of loss, did you notice any tension in your body? Did you have to put the book down and step away? Did you feel eager to keep reading, though in the past you may have been repelled by the words on the page? Some may find it difficult to connect to any strong feelings right after loss. Others may notice that they are not truly numb, but actively turning emotions off when they begin to bubble under the surface. The most common worry I hear from people who have not yet begun to sit with their loss is that if they take the lid off their grief, they'll never be able to put it back on. It is scary to think that we could be forever consumed and immobilized by grief. However, if we never take the lid off, grief will ooze out through the cracks and the lid will take itself off—often in ways that we don't like. By slowly twisting the lid and releasing some of the pressure, you can begin to practice being with the feelings as they arise and building trust in your ability to do so.

Cognitively: Updating Your Inner GPS

After loss, along with traversing new emotional terrain, there is cognitive terrain that you might struggle to navigate. In 2014, three neuroscientists were awarded the Nobel Prize for their groundbreaking contribution to the discovery of grid cells in the brain. In one study, they recorded the neural firing of a rat as it made daily visits to a box. After the box's landmark feature, a LEGO tower, was removed, the rat's neural firing persisted for approximately five days when it was in the area where the tower previously stood. Essentially, this study showed that we have an internal map, or GPS, that takes time to update. Psychologist Mary Frances O'Connor shows how this connects to grief in her book *The Grieving Brain* (2022). She likens life after loss to walking in the dark. We expect that our loved ones will be in the next room because that's where they have always been. This is how radically loss rewires us, showing how vital it is that you give yourself grace in your process and its timing. You are learning to exist in a body that doesn't yet know how to be without your loved one.

Relationally: Variation in Family Response

Grief is rarely an entirely solitary experience. As losses tend to be shared, grief is often collective. This can mean that we mourn alongside each other or that our grief bumps up against another's, creating tension.

One expectation that can quickly be upturned after loss is that each member of a family or community will have a similar reaction to the same death. It may feel like everyone should respond to the loss of this one person in the same way. However, the truth is that individuals are inherently unique, relationships between two individuals are unique, and each loss is unique—therefore, so is the grief. Though there is an opportunity to come together around a shared loss, variations in responses to it can give rise to misunderstandings and resentments, which may move grievers apart.

Grief reactions fall into two broad categories: there tend to be those who go toward it and those who move away from it. You may be a person who wishes to face the depth of the loss head on, but find yourself in a group that struggles to do so. Recognizing this dynamic (we'll talk through how to navigate it in chapter 6) is a helpful first step on what will be a longer journey of determining where family can come together, where it feels like forcing connection, and where it becomes necessary to seek support in alternate spaces.

Relationally: Receiving the Grief of Others

Amid all this, you are expected to face the outside world for funeral services. If this feels like a blur, it would be understandable why. Not only is this an event that places symbols of finality on the loss, you are effectively hosting a gathering to receive the sorrows of others. It may feel as though this event is less designed for your process or memorializing your person, and more for others' sense of closure—to make their death more real—something you may already feel starkly. However, if you lost your person during the height of COVID-19, you may have experienced an added grief from not being able to gather. For some, this part of the loss is a celebration of life, and for others, it is just an event to get through until you can get back home and into pajamas. There is no right or wrong way to experience your loved one's service.

What the Beginning of Grief Isn't For

If you are no longer in the early days of your grief, do you remember analyzing or trying to change your experience as you were having it? Do you remember feeling any pressure to immediately create meaning from your loss? Consider whether these efforts helped or caused more hurt. What would you communicate to that earlier version of yourself now, if you could?

If you are in the beginning and some of these parts of early grief sound familiar, you may be wondering what to do with them. First, I would encourage you to refrain from doing a few things. Here is what the beginning is *not* for.

No Analyzing or Trying to Change

Your job right now is not to analyze your feelings or experiences, nor to try to change them. Many people—especially those who identify as perfectionists, caretakers, eldest children, and the "strong" friends—struggle with trying to figure it all out too quickly, wanting, understandably, to avoid the pain. This is how we keep healing work on a superficial level, leaving the real stuff to surface later on. We can't intellectualize our way out of grief. We can only feel our way *through* it. What if I told you there is nothing that you have to change about what you're experiencing? When you need to support yourself through the moments when feelings become too overwhelming, I encourage you to engage in a simple grounding exercise like box breathing.

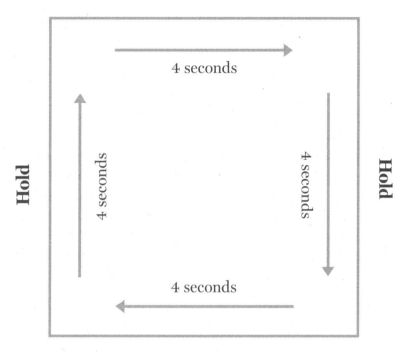

Breathe in

Hold

4 seconds

4 seconds

4 seconds

4 seconds

Hold

Breathe out

Breathe in for four seconds, hold for four, breathe out for four, hold, and so on. Repeat this four times in a row. Feel free to modify this exercise as you need. Notice what helps you feel grounded in your body.

Bear in mind that you do not need to support yourself through the moment alone. It is important, in this delicate time, to identify at least one person you can be supported by. You don't always need to know what kind of support you require—just the presence of someone who will remain flexible. Perhaps this is someone to speak with in some moments and to simply sit with in others.

Don't Force Meaning

What if I also told you that you do not need to make any meaning of this loss or its surrounding events right now? Meaning-making in grief is a delicate exploration that cannot be forced. Generally, we don't arrive at meaning anywhere near the immediate loss. Unfortunately, all too often, others attempt to bestow this upon us in the form of dreaded platitudes such as "Everything happens for a reason," and it rings hollow. Any meaning you may come to connect with your loss is only yours to find, in our own unique timeframe. If you imagine that finding meaning in this loss would feel like seeing a lighthouse upon a dark, distant shore, know that you are already on your way there by directly exploring your grief.

What the Beginning of Grief Is For

If you are seeking direction or relief in this moment, here is the part you have been waiting for, although it may be more subtle than you were expecting. This is what you can do, right now.

Surviving

This time, the very beginning of grief, is for survival. Going through the movements of daily life, which once felt second nature, may feel more like walking on stilts, with the awkward coordination of a newborn animal. In some ways, life has completely started over, so this is a time to recalibrate the expectations you set for yourself. We will begin working on this in the next chapter.

Noticing Feelings

To the extent that you are able, I encourage you to begin practicing mindfulness of your emotions. Much of what I hope to support you with is this: To accept your feelings and more sustainably be with them. There is no secret formula that will result in the eradication of your emotions, nor would you want (I imagine) to be fully without them. The goal is to allow what you are feeling to surface enough that you can fully grieve. When what you are noticing becomes overwhelming, return to a grounding exercise like box breathing. I will be right here.

Final Thoughts

Whether sudden or anticipated, grief is multidimensional, impacting your mind, body, and spirit. If you are in the aftermath right now, all you need to do is observe. If you are looking back, all you need to do is recall what you can about the initial impact that loss had on you. Next, we'll begin looking at your survival, together.

REFLECTION QUESTION

Which emotions feel easiest or safest to identify and be with? Which feel the hardest and least safe?

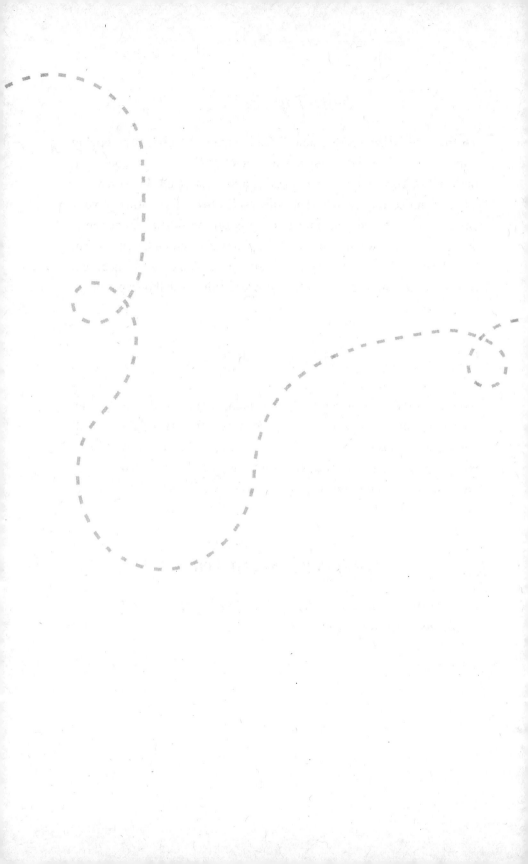

CHAPTER 3

Survival Mode

"How are you doing, Alex?" My aunt would ask me over weekly dinners after piano lessons.

"I'm fine, I'm busy," I'd reply, very assuredly for a nine year old.

After the loss of my father, my mother signed me up for a plethora of extracurricular activities and followed behind with a folding chair. I carried on my father's busy energy, guided by some instinct to fill my time. In contrast, the weeks following the loss of my mother were a slow, heavy daze—a physical collapse in which I was finally able to sleep, even when I was awake. I had nothing to watch out for anymore because the big, bad thing had already happened. The nightmare had been realized. Life as I knew it was over, so my living had to pause.

At first, existence can feel so unbearable that we grasp at anything that will help. We may not be reaching to feel "good" yet—just stabilizing our internal system with enough soothing to keep going. I grasped at little comforts where I could find them from within the confines of my grief cocoon: I listened to a ton of '80s music and looked at pictures of my mother, mostly from that era. Like a sponge, I soaked up any information I could about her earlier life to stay close to her. Yet it was like remembering someone else. Initially, this was all I could really do. Immediately after these losses, all I had the capacity for was survival.

And survival looked vastly different with each loss. How we survive the early days of grief is unique to each person and through every loss we face.

Before continuing, I acknowledge that you may be reading this from survival mode or from a later vantage point in your grief. If you fall into the latter, I encourage you to still read these pages. If you are not in the very early days of loss, here is how to use this chapter. Cast your mind back to the beginning and ask yourself the following:

- What did those early days look like?

- What sorts of thoughts was I having?

- What support did I receive?

- What got me through?

If it is difficult to remember, that makes sense. Grieving people tend to shift into autopilot when their pain is at its most raw, automatically and unconsciously slipping inside a protective bubble. Remember these questions and any reflections you can gather as you read.

When we enter the early days after loss, we shift into survival mode. You can think of this time as going on a personal lockdown—not thriving or living in color, just operating on our most basic settings and, even then, almost forgetting how they work. We may feel stripped of emotion, the world around us dulls, and we may not even be actively grieving—something I will discuss shortly. Or we may experience a muddy confluence of conflicting emotions and thoughts as we try to make sense of what has just happened to our lives. The early days of grief are a vortex. A place where everything is painfully real and not real at the exact same time, a place where it may be hard for others to reach us or for us to reach out.

While things felt hazy after my mother's death, I also found myself waiting for something. An underground current of anxiety asked the question: *What happens now?* After the funeral, we are in a sort of no-man's-land. This no-man's-land may feel uncharted, even if we have experienced loss before (each one is unique, after all). Also, at this point we may already begin to see people dispersing. This can make survival mode an isolating state. Hopefully, you are or were in close proximity to at least one or more supportive people during the days when you are just getting through them. Support is so vital at this time because there is emotional rawness in the early days, and loss can also manifest physically.

The Body in Survival Mode

You have maybe heard about the mind-body connection. Essentially, we cannot fully separate our emotional and physical experiences. They are intricately woven together. So, when we are emotionally pulled under into deep-sea grief, our whole bodies go too.

Hunger, Sleep, and Energy

Grief has a sneaky way of hijacking our appetites. Days after my mother's funeral, a father and daughter who lived in the neighborhood rang the doorbell with a homecooked dish. The father shared some fumbling words about the tray in his hands and the daughter made a joke about him being a Good Samaritan, rolling her eyes as teenagers do. I was floating somewhere outside of my own body, watching their whole exchange. It was so foreign, as I never had the opportunity to be annoyed with my own father. Despite their kind gesture, I didn't eat what they brought. Eating is a challenge for many people in early grief. When I could eat, my only viable source of sustenance was Top Ramen noodles. Periods of high stress and anxiety can suppress our appetites. By contrast, you may notice an increase in appetite, as certain foods become a source of comfort and the act of eating becomes a distraction. Check in with yourself here. Is nourishment an area where you could use some support?

Grief also has a way of shaping the circadian rhythm, which dictates our natural sleep cycles, not allowing us to sleep as much as we need or only allowing us to sleep and not do much else. Below the surface, our hearts and minds are trying to grasp this enormous change in our universe—even if it doesn't look like we are doing much, this is exhausting. For this reason, we may find going to sleep easier, our bodies caving to a desperate need for rest. Some may find going to sleep difficult. Remaining asleep may also be challenging. If sleep feels challenging, get settled in bed earlier than usual, and try listening to a guided meditation app. If you notice that you are not falling asleep right away, remind yourself that lying in a dark room with your eyes closed offers restoration. In this survival period, it is worth noting that a unique pang of grief happens upon waking up—a daily exercise in thundering devastation. These are moments when we think, *I almost forgot*. In the mornings, go slowly if you can, even if this means giving yourself just a few minutes to breathe before facing the world. Then, go gently.

While awake, grief casts a sluggishness over our movements that pairs with what many describe as "brain fog." Some simple actions, or all of them, previously taken for granted now feel arduous. Curling our limbs on the couch to watch a TV show—one we'll struggle to ever watch in the future because it will be tinged with the memory of these raw early days of grief—may be an act of physical exertion. If you go anywhere, perhaps to the grocery store, you might find that standing in the aisle and looking at shelves of snack foods feels incomprehensible, like you're almost not even standing there, like you're almost not even sure what you're looking at. Because how is any of this still real? You may not make it out the door for a while. However, not everyone chooses or has the option to remain so cocooned in the beginning. Getting through a day at work or parenting may feel like a welcomed distraction, an Olympic sport, or both. Making a meal, getting dressed, even showering—these actions are so commonplace that they can feel like the tiniest and starkest reminders that you are still living while they are not.

This may also be a time when we dissociate. Dissociation is considered a "defense mechanism" in which "threatening ideas and feelings are separated from the rest of the psyche" (American Psychological Association 2018). There is a spectrum of dissociating and most, if not all of us, have experienced it mildly when we daydream. Although it can be a means of pushing psychic material out in defense, it is a way of coping. By shelving our thoughts, feelings, and even sense of self, we break up some of the raw pain of grief into digestible bites over time. It can become harmful, and further support is needed when we struggle to get back into reality or feel frightened by the experience.

Research finds that it is common for bereaved people to report a range of physical concerns including headaches, stomach upset, and dizziness (Konkolÿ Thege et al. 2012). Grief has even been linked with inflammation in the body (Fagundes et al. 2019). New health challenges can arise in the wake of loss, so try to practice mindfulness and not overlook any potential medical needs you may have. You may require more holistic care than talk-therapy alone can provide, including healing modalities like breathwork, meditation, and gentle movement. It is vital to know the scope of grief's impact—what you are feeling in your body is real and yes, to go on with life really is this hard. Engaging in the daily tasks of living in survival mode can feel like climbing a mountain. We may find that what our bodies do easily, however, is reach for the ones we have lost.

Muscle Memory

It happens without notice or your permission: You think to tell them something and reach for your phone. Maybe you even type in their name, prepared to write a message or call their number. There have been innumerable instances just like this one, except this time, you realize that they are not alive on the other end to answer. A hot flash of agony strikes as you jolt into remembering.

Our people reside in our muscle memory. Especially in the beginning, we experience automatic impulses to reach out, over and over, until we learn and adapt to this seemingly impossible new reality. These moments may arise further down the line, but less frequently and automatically, becoming less of a reflex and more of a wish. From your place of survival, you may feel as though you are taking baby steps forward, thinking, *Ah, okay, I could breathe today*. Then you reach to call them, and are rendered incapacitated once again. In these moments, I would like you to remind yourself that you are not going backward. Say to yourself: *I am adapting to the impossible*.

Reframing Resilience

The way that you talk to yourself throughout your grief, especially when you are just trying to survive it, truly matters. More often than not, I find that the grieving give themselves little credit for their ability to get through. When we allow ourselves to see that grief changes everything, then the fact that loss brings life to a halt makes sense. It is necessary to see and believe in your own resilience. Every day you are rising to meet an extraordinary challenge, and you deserve to recognize your strength (even if you don't feel strong).

What is Resilience?

Resilience is a word we hear often, sometimes dreading it or taking it in without stopping to consider what it actually means. Merriam-Webster dictionary defines resilience as "the capability of a strained body to recover its size and shape after deformation caused especially by compressive stress" (2024). For our purposes, consider that the pain of loss pushes in all around us, leaving us crumpled. By letting grief transform us, we discover that we won't ever return to the same exact shape we were before. Instead, we can expand little by little, slowly recovering in size, making room for both sorrow and even joy. A second definition of *resilience* offered in the dictionary is "an ability to recover from or adjust easily to misfortune or change." This may be aligned with your idea of resilience, particularly the notion of "easily" recovering. What do you picture when the word comes to mind? Perhaps something grand or heroic, even. The kind of resilience you embody in the dark days of your grief may be much softer, quieter, and still just as present.

From the Bed to the Couch

It is essential that we reframe what resilience looks like in these early days of grief. Think of someone you deem "resilient." Consider how intimately you do, or do not, know the details of their story and how they actually got from that deep well of tragedy, up and out, into the space you see them in today. Oftentimes, we have only a vague under-standing of someone's journey. There tends to be a shadow period when the bereaved seem to disappear from view before emerging, dif-ferent, yet intact. When we are the ones inside the shadow, we may feel that others have opted to look away, or we may be self-isolating. The kind of resilience we enact largely goes unseen. We have to recognize it, first and foremost, for ourselves.

In the beginning, resilience may look like moving from the bed to the couch for the day. Later on, it may look like being hit with a grief wave and having the self-knowledge that what you need on that par-ticular day is to get back in the bed, to weep, to release, so that you can continue again. Notice how you may be creating a pathway to healing for yourself, even when the steps feel shaky. You are probably more resilient than you believe yourself to be. And, no, this does not mean that you have to go it alone.

Gathering Support

You have maybe noticed a pinch of irritation at being called "resilient." Insinuations come along with it—namely, that if you can manage to be resilient, others around you are off the hook. Maybe you imagine that resilience means you need to, or can, go it alone. It's true that much of grief processing happens on the inside. Grief is, after all, deeply personal. Yet it does not need to be carried all alone.

For some people, this is the default: to try and survive without anyone's help. If that resonates for you, consider where this comes from. Perhaps you are used to doing this or it has been the only option in the past. Consider whether it still needs to be your only option. Even the most self-sufficient people will find that grief can become too heavy to bear in isolation. Generally, people need people, regardless of resilience. It is okay to find your unique rhythm of alternating between privately tending to the most delicate parts of yourself and also seeking care and support outside of yourself. Locating just one or two people you can share some of your needs with at this point is key. It may be especially helpful if one of those people is someone who can engage with and mobilize others.

Identifying and Sharing Your Needs

You may be wondering, *But what do I need?* You may find your answer by considering what feels most difficult to do alone right now. You could be experiencing the bodily challenges of grief—difficulty sleeping, decreased appetite, or depletion of energy. Think about an area where you can let someone in, to be part of meeting the challenge. For example, say your energy is low and your appetite has been diminished, but you have a meal in mind that sounds even the slightest bit appealing. Is there someone who can prepare it for you? That way, you are able to both rest and begin welcoming some food into your body.

Hopefully you will be open to something a bit more nourishing for your system than instant noodles. But if not, I get it. I really do.

Not all needs during survival mode pertain to activities of daily living. You may also need to experience the catharsis of sharing the thoughts and feelings swirling inside of you as you grapple with another day. In addition to speaking with a friend or family member, you may even consider seeing a therapist. This choice may depend on the degree to which you feel emotionally resourced (safe and able to meet your needs) by your immediate circle's support, how comfortable you feel sharing with someone unknown to you, and how feasible it feels to get yourself to appointments.

When You Don't Know What You Need

Sometimes, we simply don't know what we need. Or we cannot locate any needs beyond the obvious. The answer, if we are being honest, is just for them to be alive. We feel the weight of that impossible need fall on us more heavily in some moments than others—and nothing else suffices. This is when we may just need to cry, sometimes on our own, sometimes in the presence of someone else. Maybe we need to be held, or have a hand to hold, or a shoulder to literally lean on. A common pitfall for people supporting us in these instances is thinking we need to hear magic words that will soothe our pain, when what is usually need is just their presence. To advocate for this, you can say something to this effect: "Don't worry about having perfect words. I'm not looking for advice in this moment. I just need to not be alone right now."

By contrast, maybe you are feeling overwhelmed by the presence of others and need to take a little more space for yourself. Consider saying, "It helps to not be alone, but sometimes I need space to be quiet with my own thoughts and feelings. Right now is one of those times." Find the words that feel right when you say them aloud to yourself.

If you are reading from the vantage point beyond grief survival, I would like to check back in on you. As you look back on those early days, how challenging was it to identify and share your needs? Did you go it alone? Did you have to? Pause to reflect, as this will be helpful to draw from later in the chapter.

Expanding Your Survival

Take into consideration what you are already doing to keep yourself afloat. It is possible to build upon your very real resilience and expand your current world, which can feel very, very small in grief. It may need to be small in the beginning. But by making your world just the tiniest bit bigger, on your own and with the support of others, you can give yourself a little more room to breathe.

I understand that when you are feeling extremely low, as though you can't get up, and someone tells you that it would really help if you went for a walk, it feels laughable, inconceivable, maybe embittering. So, if you're under the covers, I'm not going to suggest that you go for the walk yet. You can just sit up, maybe on top of the covers. Feel that. Then maybe you can stand. Feel that too. Then maybe you can go to the kitchen for a glass of water. Then maybe you can put on fresh clothes. Keep feeling what it is like to be in your body as you navigate your space. Then maybe you can go to the mailbox—but you don't need to sort through it all. Can somebody help with this? Designate them. Then perhaps you can walk around the block and come right back. You don't have to take in too much of the world around you if that is overwhelming. It may be frightening to see how little has changed. Having tunnel vision is okay, just see only what is necessary for you to safely navigate your brief path out and home. Then next time, or maybe the time after that, you can go on a longer walk.

One, Two, Three Things a Day

If it all feels too daunting, a way of getting your arms around day-to-day activities may be to start small and build upon actions of self-care incrementally. Do just one thing a day, like making coffee or tea. Then two things a day, like making coffee or tea and getting dressed. Then three things a day, like making coffee or tea, getting dressed, and going for a walk. You may need time in between each act of self-care before adding another action into the mix. One day, it may dawn on you that, without noticing, you have largely slipped out of survival mode. You will be living again.

Grief Delayed

In this chapter, you may have noticed that we are not venturing into the territory of truly grappling with the fallout of loss. There is, at this point, no analysis or call for deep introspection. Why? Grief is often delayed while we are busy surviving. This may sound like a problem to be on guard for, but it isn't. When merely existing feels like kicking into quicksand, we don't have the space to discover what our loss means or who we are now because of it. Placing temporal parameters around grief is rarely helpful. But it may give you tangible permission to know this: For many people, the first year of grief is about survival. It is a time for learning how to cope with the unthinkable, little by little. Deeper reflection and integration tend to come later, even years later, and that is okay. The repercussions of our loss and the little wisdoms of our grief often cannot be fully realized in the very early days. We need more experience living in this new reality to get there.

In the therapy room, grieving people often track time aloud, aware of a prevailing expectation that as year one of a loss comes to a close, we leave grief behind. As they hurtle over the other side of that year, they find that of course they don't move on—we never truly do. Maybe you too have thought to yourself at the one-year mark, *But I'm barely able to think about them without getting a lump in my throat.* Maybe you still find it challenging to let them cross your mind without your throat constricting and your eyes watering, during year two or three as you continue to integrate the loss. On the other end of others' expectation meter, people may be bewildered if we are not emoting at all times in the beginning. In reality, it may take time to actively and safely begin feeling again. Grief work is slow work. Recall this any time you feel pressure to speed up your process.

A Passageway, Not a Place to Stay

Hearing that you may spend a whole year just surviving may induce a sigh of relief or ring alarm bells of panic. I caution you to not bind yourself to the idea that survival equals one year. For the outside world, the first anniversary of a death is often the one that garners the most attention. It seems to be met with (often incorrect) assumptions about the amount of healing that has taken place. You are not destined to be lodged deep into the cushions of your couch for any period of time. You do have a say. And you should not have to suffer more than you already have.

Yes, survival mode is a place where we can get stuck. We tend to risk this by turning inward to the point of isolation, not reaching out for help, and not tending to the very real physical changes taking place. When we do not get these basic needs met, the absence of them doubles down on us. We remain in deep-sea grief, without even a chance to try rising to the surface and taking some breaths. Sometimes, people arrive in therapy realizing that they have spent years just surviving after loss and trauma. Perhaps they are at the surface but dog-paddling rapidly to remain afloat, their lives on hold. Anything more than surviving feels impossible. The world may feel like a terrifying place. The right supports may not have been there to make this feel less so. There is no shame in this, and it is never too late. What matters is that they have arrived at a point of readiness for more, just as you may have, or might upon finishing this book.

Final Thoughts

Survival mode is not a place to stay, and it is also not something to try and skip. Survival mode is a necessary part of contending with life-altering loss and entering it speaks to your ability to cope. It may feel less like a well-lit passage and more like a dark tunnel you wait in for an interminable amount of time, but it does lead somewhere. Survival mode is not a strange and awful exercise in deflating. It is our natural way of cocooning to insulate ourselves from the sharpness of the pain, until it becomes just bearable enough to be with. If we could teleport from the day our loved one dies to a future moment where our loss holds meaning, we would feel immense whiplash. As dull and aching as it may be, we need to pass through the in-between space. If it feels like you are in survival mode right now, you can simply credit yourself for getting through today. If you are looking back on it, ask yourself, what might you have needed that time for? How may it have ushered you, from the moment you parted with your person, to the place you are today?

Wherever you may be, remember that by recognizing your unique resilience, fostering it through incremental self-care, and identifying and expressing your needs, you are supporting yourself in the direction of living again. However, there is no rush. Grief can be exhausting, even beyond its early days, because it offers no finish line to cross. It becomes softly integrated with time, yet it lacks absolute completion. In this way, grief teaches us the practice of remaining present with ourselves in each moment. With the knowledge that there is no prize handed out for surviving most efficiently, do what you can, where you are. If you feel a strong desire to go forward, take a few steps. If you feel the magnetic pull of the couch, know that you can try again tomorrow. Next, we will look ahead toward rejoining the living world, which you may have to do while still in survival mode. Or it may come naturally as *part* of your survival, just as the childhood extracurricular activities were part of mine.

When you step out of survival mode, I invite you to do the following: Write a letter to the version of yourself that was in survival mode. Consider validating their experience and sharing where you are today. You may also wish to first write a letter from your survival-mode self to you now, giving them an opportunity to share their pain, be witnessed, and ask questions for which only you hold the answers. Finally, if all you can do right now is survive, know that is enough.

REFLECTION QUESTION

What does your resilience look like today?

CHAPTER 4

"Back to Normal"

It will be good for me to get out, we all think. I remember tagging along with a cousin for some errand. Although I don't do much at all, the errand feels like completing a triathlon. On the highway, everything appears as it usually does, and this shocks me. I am looking at things so familiar to me—yet they feel entirely alien. Or do *I* feel like an alien? Through the mental and physical fog, I gaze out the window and wonder how this world is still moving. In a matter of one week, mine has come to a complete, crashing halt.

In the car, I think about how it feels like both just a second ago and many years ago that I stood in the kitchen with my mother after she came home from an appointment with her oncologist, and she said, "We got some bad news." Her face crumpled in a way that would remain indelibly in my memory as she wrapped her arms around me. The bad news was that she had, at best, one to three months of life left. This was after a five-year journey with cancer that was at times aggressive, and at others was a slow, rocking tide of some strange normalcy. The days following this conversation were a haze of physical deterioration, final conversations, mental preparation for the absolute unpreparable—really, the impossible. In some moments, I was desperate for her suffering, as well as my anticipation of her death, to end. She would die only a week after the conversation in the kitchen.

When we hear that someone has died from cancer, we might think of words like "slow" or "expected." But her illness had become such a part of our daily lives that the nature of her death, especially with one week's notice, was jarring. Throughout her sickness, living in the moment was a skill we honed together—my mother, my sister, and I. In hindsight, my mother seemed to acknowledge that her time on Earth was coming to a close and attempted to prepare me. But I wouldn't hear of it. She was my person—the one who brought me here and was always by my side. The notion of her being anywhere else was inconceivable, unacceptable.

In the car I noticed, without anger but perhaps some irrational surprise, that the world did not freeze to acknowledge my mother's death. In real time, I was putting the jagged pieces of a painful puzzle together: Here is the world and she is no longer in it. Here is life, beating in its natural rhythm—one she is no longer contributing to—and that absence makes it seem *unnatural*. I wondered, *How do I inhabit this place without her?*

I would eventually come to find, and later help others process in my work as a therapist, this realization: After we lose someone, not only does the world keep moving, but we are expected to keep moving with it. By "moving," I mean engaging in life, socializing, going to school, running errands, returning texts, and of course, working.

WORK AFTER LOSS

The US Department of Labor states the following on their website: "The Fair Labor Standards Act (FLSA) does not require payment for time not worked, including attending a funeral. This type of benefit is generally a matter of agreement between an employer and an employee (or the employee's representative)" (2025). There is no federal law protecting bereavement leave and it is given or not given at the discretion of employers.

Take a moment to pause here and consider the following:

- How many days did you have off work?

- How was this time spent? For example, was there time built into your leave for rest or was it filled with obligations (like service planning and settling affairs) related to the loss?

- How did the time come to be agreed upon with your employer?

- Was it paid or unpaid?

- Was it enough?

For every person who reads these questions, the answers will vary. As you may have gathered by this point, variation is one of the only constants within the topic of grief. What each person experiences, needs, or finds helpful will be different.

Rejoining the Living World

In the immediate aftermath of loss, it can feel as though we are shrouded in a fog, suspended somewhere murky between our old lives and the ongoing lives of others. It's normal to feel disconnected from our sense of self, our bodies, and other people as we sit with the unimaginable, still in survival mode. At some point, we are called to rejoin the living world. You might notice that this call comes from within—a desire to feel like yourself or lean into parts of what now feels like an old life. You might hear, loud and clear, the call coming from outside you, perhaps from work, family, or friends. The call compels us to cross a bridge from surviving to living, or at least what looks like living. For a time, it may feel like you are going through the motions, imitating the appearance of what it means to live, without truly feeling it.

There are many bridges to the living world that we are encouraged, maybe urged, or even pushed, to cross. Work is a bridge, school is a bridge, caretaking is a bridge. Anything that prods us to leave the confines of our early grief cocoon and paves some ground in front of us to walk on, is a bridge. I often hear people in this part of their grief say that they are just trying to "put one foot in front of the other." Though it might sound like a cliché, that seemingly or formerly intuitive action of moving forward can now feel treacherous. Loss shatters the ground beneath us, sending us on a freefall with no defined landing. What once felt certain no longer does.

Why We Fear Crossing the Bridge

For many, the bridge is a dreaded place. You might feel that you cannot rise to the occasion of being out *there*. It feels daunting and, maybe on the darker days, it feels utterly pointless. Let's look more closely at these feelings and try to understand them better. When we are inactive right after loss, we can stay suspended in the in-between—a place that can feel comforting at best and at the very least, neutral. When we step out, interacting with people and places that once felt familiar, though our new reality is anything but, we are put in direct contact with the truth that our loved one is absent in an ongoing world. With the bright, hot pain of loss already so fresh, why would we want to bring ourselves any closer to such reminders? It is an understandable question.

Much of what makes it challenging to stay on the bridge, and not turn back once we have taken a few steps, is the experience or imagined experience of conversing with others. In particular, you might feel unease anticipating that your grief may not be known. Perhaps you are going into a space where you will be speaking with people who are unaware that you have just gone through a major loss. This often raises the question of whether or not to share.

Among the many clients I have worked with, this seems to boil down, like so many facets of walking with loss, to personal choice. I tend to hear scenarios in which the other—an acquaintance, colleague, or relative stranger out in the world—asks a question and the answer involves disclosing the loss. The question might be about family, how you spent a holiday, or something as broad and unanswerable as how you have been. For a moment, the options hang in the air: Do you skirt the piece of the question that connects to your loss? You could. Do you acknowledge that piece head-on? You could. I feel for us grievers in these moments because over time, we come to know them so well.

At some point in my journey, I started to notice how these conversations would take a turn, but my conversational partner wouldn't be aware of it. They did not yet know that they were steering us into waters that were uncharted for them, familiar for me, and potentially awkward for us both. For example, I was asked, "How do your parents handle that?" *They don't.* I used to inwardly grimace and land on some semblance of acknowledgment: "Actually, they're not alive." There was something about saying "not alive" that felt less disastrous, as though it did not mean the same thing as "dead." I tended to use language that was more palatable in an effort to comfort the other person, fearful of burdening them—a subject I'll discuss in chapter 6. What I want to highlight here is how this sort of mental gymnastics, which you may or may not find yourself doing, is taxing.

Let's say you are entering a space where people do know about your loss. You may imagine, perhaps with good reason, that the possibility of grief spilling out will not be well-received. After all, it usually only takes one or two encounters with the outside world, sometimes starting at the funeral, to notice that many people seem uncomfortable in the presence of grief or even at the mere mention of death and loss. You might have been primed for this in your family of origin, if vulnerability and emotions were considered taboo. When first venturing out, there are all of these anticipations and assumptions (though hopefully, there may be some pleasant surprises), and there are so many unknowns. This can all feel quite scary: *How will I feel? How will I show up? Will I seem as different as I am on the inside? How will others respond to me? What is going to happen?* The truth is that you simply won't know until you are there.

It may be helpful to start processing the fact that you are likely beginning to sense internal changes. At its core, internal changes are what make the bridge to the living world feel so shaky. You are on the precipice of a transformation that perhaps doesn't feel coherent or cohesive yet, so you can't put words to it. You certainly don't recognize this life that you're in or feel like "you" anymore, yet you may feel expected to continue being the "you" others have always known and fit into your life as you always have. Contrary to those expectations, research on bereavement has cited "identity disturbance" as central to long-term grief management (Harris et al. 2021), which we'll explore more together in later chapters. We know ourselves, in large part, through our relationships. So when we lose someone significant to us, as the ground beneath us shatters, our self-knowing may become less clear. *How do I inhabit this place without her?* expands to *Who am I without her?* It is completely natural to feel uncertain about how to communicate the ongoing shifts that move through you as you grapple with existential questions and wonder whether this transforming version of yourself will be welcomed or not.

So, what happens when we put all these fears together? They form a mosaic of supermonster anxiety. You step into a landscape that, despite looking "normal," feels anything but. You may be squarely confronted with the potentially unchanged expectations of others, and risk feeling emotionally wrought and treated less gently than at home. This is the part where I encourage you to take a deep breath. What we have been sitting with is the fear, not the facts. Fear that: is fairly well-informed (yes, our society largely turns away from and misunderstands grief); scans your environment and concludes this life is no longer trustworthy; is merely trying to protect you in a softened, vulnerable state. Each time the fear swells, I encourage you to meet it, acknowledge it, and name it. Consider what fear is attempting to provide for you. You may even want to thank it for an earnest attempt. *I see what you are trying to do for me but there is only so much anticipation I can engage in before I take some steps to rejoin the world.* By treating the fear like a well-intended but overeager companion, you can begin to create some space from it.

Why We Cross the Bridge Nonetheless

The call to cross the bridge remains, despite our fears. For many, there is little choice but to heed it. Keeping yourself or your family afloat financially often provides the most powerful push out of the grief cocoon. This may mean less contemplation about what it will feel like. If you do have a degree of choice about when to return to work, you may notice yourself reluctantly crossing the bridge in response to an external pressure that whispers *move on*. People may not use those words directly. Instead, they may ask when you plan to return to your job and other obligations, even immediately after the loss. Returning may be proposed as a helpful action you can take—but the nuance that it is both necessary and difficult is lost. To assess when it's time, first check in with how it feels to take care of yourself at home, how your current level of interpersonal interaction is feeling (are you ready for more?), and how your job typically makes you feel. A sense of purpose might be helpful.

You may even welcome and find relief in the call to continue on. Some opt out of time off altogether and carry on with previously held plans for travel, courses, or social gatherings. Perhaps this describes you: Loss has upended your life. The events that have occurred, the feelings swelling inside of you—you have had no say in any of it, you have given no permission. Your job is right there, waiting inside your computer, and all you need to do is send an email sharing that you'll be back on Monday. You'll be back, as in your body will be back in the office. Perhaps laced into your message, there is a subconscious wish— *I'll be back, the me I've always been. I can still be me.* This is when crossing the bridge to the living world can provide great relief. We may crave some sense of agency or normalcy, and therefore be eager to grasp onto anything that might offer it. Perhaps as a caretaker to a loved one who was dying, you felt completely out of control, but in your work life you feel capable and certain. Stepping back into a familiar environment and still feeling a sense of belonging there could reassure you—*I can still live.*

Often, it does not feel exactly the same. I caution you to be mindful that in your quest for a life raft of stability, you do not overlook the depth of your pain and the changes it is bringing. It is helpful to not remain stagnant after loss *and*, at the same time, forcing an old "normal" instead of observing what feels challenging is a sure way to suppress your emotions. It is also helpful to remain mindful of the supports around you.

How Others Help and Hurt

How others respond to us as we start to navigate a daily life without our person can have a considerable effect on how equipped we feel to keep showing up. I have seen pressure make a difference for my clients through its presence, absence, and intensity—whether self-inflicted pressure, pressure from others, or a combination of both. When we receive the pressure that pushes us along, connoting a lack of understanding that our life is entirely different now, we may feel more isolated. We may think we are not doing this "right." In an effort to reduce feelings of isolation or shame, we run the risk of moving into daily routines or spaces sooner than feels right for us. The inauthenticity embedded in this choice makes itself known eventually. We might become physically rundown and fatigued, emotionally overwhelmed, or both.

If others convey an understanding that we may feel scared to rejoin the living world after loss, that world becomes the slightest bit more approachable. In grief, we mostly need to be seen. Those seeking to support loved ones who have met great loss should know that gentle encouragement that acknowledges the enormity of what they are experiencing aids healing in authentic and sustainable ways. Acting as though it is *not so bad* rarely does the trick.

Despite my teenaged insecurity about feeling known among my peers for being orphaned, the fishbowl aspect of the small community I grew up in was not all bad. In retrospect, I was afforded support that only a small community with many eyes could provide. It was a support approach that many could learn from. At some point after my mother died, my guidance counselor and principal, who were in communication with my sister and aunt, came over one morning to talk. "Tell us what you need," they said. After a couple of weeks off school, I returned slowly, incrementally, a few class periods at a time. Throughout this time, they sensed the gravity and finality of being left parentless, without having to live it. They anticipated that I would have new needs, without assuming what they would be. They showed compassion for my complex situation. Quite literally, they showed up, and with coffee. I will never forget their thoughtfulness for my impending walk out onto the bridge. Their support, along with family members who were eager to collaborate, helped me to support myself and, to this day, support others.

Now What?

Though much is unknown about how you will experience the world without your person who died, there are ways that you can prepare. These suggestions are intended to provide you with a safety net, something to catch you when it all becomes too much and you need a soft place to land. Just as I was provided with preparations for my return to the living world, I would like to offer these to you.

Go at Your Pace: My ability to take a break from school and then gradually return was a privilege that is not afforded to all, though it should be. Within the realistic bounds of what is available to you, or what can be made available to you through self-advocacy, what pace feels right for you? Notice that I am not asking what pace you can manage to go at. I am also not encouraging you to go unnecessarily slowly. As a unique grieving individual, you may find it genuinely anchoring to return to the familiar on the sooner side.

Self-Advocate: As the person going through the loss, consider setting the tone—others may follow your cues. Imagine that perhaps others won't know what to expect, rather than assuming that they have specific expectations. Keep your sense of your own pacing in mind so that, if you do encounter any expectations, you can communicate this. Ask yourself: *Who needs to be aware of my needs? Who needs to understand me?* Each answer may vary. For instance, you may need certain people in your life to be aware of boundaries you are setting (like the amount of time you take for bereavement or activities you won't participate in as you grieve). But you only need one or two very close support people to truly understand the *why* behind these boundaries. There is, of course, always the chance that your self-advocacy will be judged and even pressed upon. In these instances, grief and its transformative nature becomes an exercise in loosening our grip on others' perceptions of us.

Have an Exit Plan: Taking breaks sustains us as we navigate the world after loss. When I returned to school after my mother died, it was not only incremental but also came with an understood plan that if I needed a break, I could go to the guidance counselor's office or the nurse's station. If I needed to go home, I could do that too. In your day-to-day life, where are the soft spaces you can retreat to? How might you sense that you need to retreat there? Is there anyone in your life who you would like to have join you in that place? I encourage you to write your answers to these questions somewhere you can easily reference.

Give Yourself Grace: I trust that someone, perhaps you, will read the words in this section suggesting that it is okay to go at your pace, to self-advocate, to take breaks, and think: *Sure, that's nice*, then consciously or subconsciously intend to disregard the advice. If that is the case, I gently invite you to read this section again. There is nothing that I need to know about you and your particular circumstances in order to freely offer a strong suggestion that you show yourself compassion. I assure you that the words on this page are not written for someone else out there. They are written for you.

What Helps About Being in the World

You may ask: *Why put myself in the crosshairs of a painful reality?* The short answer is that it's worth it. In early grief, the numb coating of survival mode is often what we need, but if we stay there rather than wading out to actively engage with our grief, we miss out on truly living. To begin, we have to decide that we don't want to miss out. If that feels too far out of reach, that is okay. Take small steps first and decide along the way.

People who are grieving not only find it challenging to reenter the terrain of life after loss, but also to stay engaged in it. It is not necessarily a matter of going to work once and then feeling integrated back into the world. If only. We may show up where we need to be, play a part, and stay withdrawn in other areas—not keeping connected with friends, for instance. With too much time suspended in the in-between, we may ruminate in the depths of despair and risk cementing thoughts like these as truths: *I'm never going to feel joy again; Things are hopeless.* We know from research that decreasing participation in living reduces access to experiences that would actually refute those beliefs (Eisma et al. 2020). Only by taking the risk of going out there can we access a reality in which joy and hope are still possible for us.

Being out in the world also serves another function—grief integration. When we withdraw from life (including social time and work), we prevent ourselves from having experiences that cause us to meet the painful reality of our loved one's absence. This thwarts the challenging but necessary task of integrating the loss into our new and emerging sense of self (Eisma et al. 2020). The more we avoid, the more we struggle with internal dissonance, finding ourselves stuck between our old life and the one that is surfacing. Confronting the painful reality isn't about needlessly suffering. It isn't about getting locked into a place of sadness from which we cannot escape. It is about letting the pain surface enough that we can use it to find a way through.

Loss and grief call upon us to stretch, adapt, and reconfigure our sense of identity like nothing else in this life. The experience asks us to write a new story about what this life is, what it looks like, what it feels like, and maybe even someday, what it means. By doing so, we mindfully carve out a path that makes our ongoing life feel worth living, while not overlooking or severing our connection to the person we lost.

Greeting new and unfamiliar parts of ourselves may also lead us to the conclusion that there are changes we need to make to our daily lives (such as our values, how we spend our time, and who we spend time with). Loss has reconfigured us on a molecular level and now we need the rhythms and routines of life to shift with us. This is not a homework assignment to be completed overnight, but a slow uncovering that can only be done by feeling—as painful as it is—life without the physical presence of someone we deeply love. I won't pretend that the benefits of leaving your comfort zone, integrating the reality of loss, and finding a way to continue will be immediate. They are an outcome that you will find over time and feel more fully in the long-term.

Final Thoughts

When we start to rejoin the world after loss, we don't simply go "back to normal." It is essential to reframe our understanding of this. With the loss of someone so vital to our lives, the whole landscape shifts—even if upon first glance, everything still looks the same. Grief does send us on a freefall, but perhaps eventually we do experience a sense of having landed, albeit somewhere else entirely. In Victor Fleming's *The Wizard of Oz* movie (1939), Dorothy's house goes up in the twister just after she is knocked unconscious—for our purposes, an analog to the early fog of grief in which time is incomprehensible. Her home spins, as we do in the turmoil of discovering that life as we *know* it can quickly become life as we *knew* it. As the house begins to descend, she awakens, clinging to her levitating bed. After landing with a harsh thud on the ground and glancing around her room, Dorothy opens the door to find that she is somewhere unfamiliar (you know the line). Everything transforms from sepia to technicolor. In grief, we know this to occur in reverse. Upon opening the door, everything is in black and white. It is only by venturing out into the world, moving into this unfamiliar version of life at a tempo only we can hear within us, that hue by hue, the color fades back in.

REFLECTION QUESTION

If you tune out the noise of dominant culture, what do you believe about the timing of your process?

CHAPTER 5

Riding the Waves

It's my dad's birthday today. I'm not entirely sure how old he would be, but I know that in my lifetime, he has been absent for more of his birthdays than he was present. I have been acutely aware of March 27th inching closer on the calendar, but it hasn't occurred to me that any preparation would be needed. I'm at my office when a text from my sister arrives: *I know I've told you before, but I don't know if you remember that dad used to say he hoped you'd listen to "You'll Never Walk Alone" from the movie* Carousel. *I'm listening to it now.*

My father wanted to ensure that I wouldn't forget him or, if I did, I would be comforted by the lyrics. I immediately duck into the privacy of the bathroom with my headphones. My eyes sting as I listen to the song because *here he is*. How could I ever forget? Of course, there is no forgetting anyone who is such a part of you. Even though I was young when he died, I possess a deep knowing of him. Most of my memories are sensorial rather than rooted in conversation: The scents of Banana Boat tanning oil, Keri Lotion, and Windex. The first fizzy sip of a Coke and the sensation of towels laid down on hot leather car seats after a day at the beach. Copious amounts of hair gel under my little hands while he let me play "hairdresser" on his salt and pepper head.

The steadiness of Saturday errands to the bank (where I get a lollipop), Kristina's convenience store (where I get a slush if it's summertime), the car wash, dry cleaners, grocery store, and sometimes Toody's restaurant for meatballs and sauce. The images of smiling faces and sounds of kind exchanges because he seems to know everyone. The vision of him at our pool, opening the cover, testing it with those little strips while I hope for the right color, skimming it, diving into it, and letting me pick him up and carry him around in the water to feel strong. The swell of pride in "helping" him open the video store for the day. The feeling of inexplicable desperation to one day need braces and borrowing his gold chain to hold them across my teeth and pretend. The sound of him on the phone calling various stores to find the *right* doll and the knowledge, later, that he crossed state lines to get it. Just the right stimuli in my environment can transport me back to being in his presence. So no, I haven't forgotten. Yet, I've certainly tried not to feel.

For many years, the days and weeks leading up to my parents' death anniversaries and birthdays involved a mix of ignoring and bracing for impact, keeping my fingers crossed that my emotions would be kept at bay. I don't fault previous versions of myself for trying to resist grief. It's painful, unfixable, and frowned upon by our dominant culture. There is an unspoken nudge to feel less and less with each passing year. If anything, though, we may feel more and more as the years go by and we encounter new ways to miss them.

Grief Waves: The Basics

What I experienced in my office bathroom was a grief wave. Almost all grieving people experience them. There is a reason the adage "grief comes in waves" has stuck around. It is, in my estimation, the closest phrase for capturing what happens as we live with loss. Grief waves are essentially swells of emotion and physical sensation. We may feel more acute sadness, longing, disbelief, or even anger. We might notice tension or exhaustion in our bodies, finding ourselves needing more rest than usual. These waves can occur around significant dates or milestones, as well as on ordinary days, in grocery stores and while doing laundry and in the midst of a movie—almost anywhere and in any situation you can imagine. I know what you might be thinking: *So, basically they can happen at any time?*

The most important thing to keep in mind as we dive further into grief waves is that they are supposed to happen. They are not a defect, or a sign of dysfunction, and they usually do not signal a crisis. If anything, a grief wave highlights our ability to adapt to life's deepest pains and most tender challenges. Think about it like this: At some point after loss, you are able to go about daily life, not only functioning but maybe even experiencing joy. (If you are not there yet, that's okay.) From time to time, you need to give yourself space to pause and feel into the depth of what you have gone through, coming into closer contact with what you always know to be true on some level: your person has really died and it does really hurt that much. The wave is a deep and visceral remembering. It is when all that remains under the surface rises up. The grief has never disappeared, it has just slipped into the background while you were living. We live, we grieve, we rest, repeat. This is how we grow through grief.

Triggers and Coping Strategies

Grief waves can go on for just a few moments and can span as long as a few days. They may start slowly ahead of a significant date. This is an especially important time to seek out support and not isolate. It can also be vitally helpful to understand what tends to bring the grief up. So, what triggers a grief wave?

Milestone Events

In the text exchange with my sister on my father's birthday, I lamented being flooded with tears at my workplace. *I don't know why this is hurting me so much this year, I guess all the good things happening,* I surmised. It wasn't just his birthday that triggered my grief, it was also the presence of so many exciting changes in my life. I was planning my wedding, which would take place that summer and then I would be off to graduate school. One might think that these milestones would provide a buffer from the sadness and longing, or at least a welcome distraction. The truth is, however, that the good days hurt too.

This might sound like: *I thought I had worked through this. I just don't know how I'm going to do it without them. It's obviously not going to look like I had pictured.* Milestones are often the entry point for grief therapy. The death itself can certainly be the catalyst to seeking support, however in many cases the joyful events (like marriages, births, moves, career changes) that come later often inspire us to reach out. This is where our dominant culture pushes back, suggesting that if the loss was not recent and good things are happening, it's well past time to stop grieving. Statements I tend to share in response, which simply hold a mirror to the reality, include: *You may have processed the loss and it's time for a reintegration. Of course, you don't know how you're going to do it without them. It makes sense that this is not what you had pictured.* Milestones activate grief waves because in their midst, we are not able to hear our person's unique words of encouragement, or their expressions of pride or excitement for us. The realization that we cannot share the good days with them brings renewed grief.

One way of easing the shock of a landmark moment or event without our person who died is to intentionally carry them with us. This could look like displaying a photo of them at your wedding venue, baby shower, going away party, or new work desk. It could also look like wearing a garment or piece of jewelry they owned. No material items are even necessary. Carrying them into the milestone in ways that ease the harshness of a grief wave, may include speaking about them with someone who is physically present.

Birthdays

Throughout the year, there are dates on the calendar that hold weight and bring our loss to the forefront. Your birthday or the birthday of your person who died can understandably bring up grief and give a whole new meaning to the "birthday blues." If your person's birthday is coming up, you may find yourself dreading an otherwise happy day. Not only are you confronted with the reality that you do not get to celebrate them as you may have in years past, most cruelly, they are not getting another year older. There is a unique kind of math that the grieving do here, calculating how old their loved one would be while simultaneously holding the image of that person at the age they were when they passed. We wonder what their lives would have looked like, what they would have looked like, what our life would be like, if they were here growing alongside us. Anger and a sense of injustice can bubble up as we do so. Of course it does. Their not being here feels and is plainly, simply wrong.

When it comes time for our own birthday, we may not feel up for celebrating or even acknowledging the day in any way. We may again engage in grief counting—refreshing ourselves on how old we were when they died and how old we are now. Birthdays can be gut-wrenching because the person who may have celebrated us the most, perhaps our partner, friend, or sibling is no longer present to do so. For those who have lost a parent, birthdays can feel much more existential than usual, highlighting the absence of one of the only other people present at the moment you came into the world.

There is no right or wrong way to live through a birthday after loss. However much or little celebrating you do, is your choice. If you feel compelled to honor your person's birthday (or honor them on your own birthday) in some way, think back to their favorite foods, activities, places, even movies—anything that feels like them. Pick one: a meal to make, a hobby to engage in, a place to go, a film to watch. Consider whether you would like to do this honoring on your own or in community. Ask yourself who you may want to be with on the day and let them know ahead of time. If this feels like a daunting commitment to make, ask if they can be available and flexible if you decide you are not up for it when the time comes. Embracing your person's favorites is a way to connect with them and this connection can anchor you through a wave. Yes, these activities may bring up tearfulness. Remember that the goal is not to feel less. It is to feel *through*.

Death Anniversaries

In my parent loss therapy groups, participants commonly share when their parents' death anniversaries are, particularly if they are going to occur during the ten weeks that we share space. It can feel like a sacred piece of information that we wish to give others about where we are headed. A common theme we process is how a whole season can be tinged with loss and anticipation, as a slow wave of dread creeps through one or two months. Sometimes, the anticipation can even feel more intense than the day itself.

People tend to assume that the greater the number of years that have passed, the less painful the loss. However, anniversaries can sharpen the edges of grief because they highlight the passage of time. Here is a reframe you can use to validate your own grief and explain this to someone in your life who may not understand: Yes, over time we may adapt more to life without them *and* the more time goes by, the harder we can be struck by the painful realization that it has been *that* long since we last saw our person.

We tend to feel more somber on death anniversaries than birthdays and there is even less of a roadmap for how to approach them.

Each year, the death anniversary of the person you lost will likely differ in terms of how you feel and what you need. It is completely natural to experience the wave of grief more acutely, or conversely be more distracted based on what is going on in the rhythm of your life. When and if you feel compelled to acknowledge the day through action, here are some ritual ideas to help you honor the significance of the date or self-soothe. Note that these activities are not exclusive to death anniversaries. Perhaps there is a different day of the year or a certain holiday you have particular difficulty moving through. Consider trying any of the following:

Visiting: Be with them however you can. This may include going to their burial place or the site where their ashes were scattered. It may involve going to any location that makes you feel close to them. While there, sit in peaceful silence, write to them, or speak to them—aloud or in your mind.

Embracing Your Favorites: Engage in self-care and treat yourself by leaning into what feels good. Check in with yourself and consider if the "favorite" you are leaning toward is a healthy coping mechanism or not. One helpful metric for this is to consider whether there are any negative side effects or consequences. Call in compassion for yourself if you feel drawn to self-destructive behaviors and plan to reach out to a trusted support person or resource.

Carrying Out an Act of Kindness: Honor your person by doing something kind for someone else, whether a friend, family member, or a stranger. This can be as simple as holding a door for someone. Perhaps there is an organization you feel compelled to donate to, one your person supported or appreciated. Engaging an act of kindness can naturally increase serotonin, dopamine, and oxytocin, which are neurotransmitters responsible for well-being, reward, and pleasure. This chemical boost may help, even just a little, to carry you through or restore you after a wave.

Tending to Your Physical Body: It has thankfully become main-stream knowledge that our lived experience shows up in our physical vessels. Grief, which often overlaps with trauma, can create tension and a sense of being weighed down in our bodies. Offer your body extra support by engaging in gentle movement, taking a bath or a long shower, or receiving a massage.

Creating an Altar: Whether you are spiritual or not, one way you can honor the anniversary of a loved one's death is by creating space for them in your home. In a visible spot, arrange candles, flowers, photos of them, and other meaningful objects. Set this altar up for the day or let it maintain permanent residence in your space. More on this in chapter 8.

Writing a Letter to Them: While visiting a sacred place or spending time by your altar, privately write a letter. What you include is entirely yours to decide. You can consider sharing reflections on the past year, any feelings that are coming up for you, or any questions you may be grappling with. After, you can save it or carefully burn it. More on this in chapter 9.

Gathering and Sharing: If being alone on the anniversary feels like it may veer from solitude into loneliness, consider who you may want to spend time with as you remember your person. Ahead of the date, discuss this and plan to set aside time to come together. Maybe you meet to talk over dinner, maybe you connect virtually or via a phone call. Speak about memories you feel called to share and ask if they will share some of their own.

The Everyday

Joan Didion wrote that grief can "obliterate the dailiness of life" (2005). I think all of us have felt that sense of obliteration at one point or another, perhaps even when we were least expecting it. The truth is that not all grief waves abide by a calendar and, really, time is a strange beast when it comes to loss. Some triggers present as stirring and poignant moments within ordinary circumstances. I was with friends downtown in a sticky basement bar, amidst a sea of yelling footy devotees, watching a Liverpool game on TV. If you are, by chance, a Liverpool FC fan, you likely know what I am about to share. At the game's close, the team, people in the stands, and everyone in the bar broke into song. *That* song, "You'll Never Walk Alone." It is the team's anthem, and I had no idea. A lump formed in my throat and my vision got blurry. This time, I knew why and I didn't push it away. Instead, I let myself feel through those moments while the voices bellowed around me. If anyone noticed, I must have looked like the deepest-feeling fan in the room.

In the ordinariness of day-to-day life, we may also feel struck by a sharp remembrance of all that has changed for us: seeing friends doubled over in laughter at an inside joke, witnessing a couple bicker on the street, hearing a mother and daughter deliberate in a dressing room. These are moments when I often hear self-judgment come up for clients as they say, "It shouldn't be a big deal." We tend to expect that a significant date is going to trigger a grief response and this feels justifiable. But when grief comes up during seemingly benign moments in the wild, we might feel less patient with ourselves. The times when we feel less able to access patience are precisely when we need to give ourselves more self-compassion. You are out in the world being a person without your person. It is a big deal.

Grief Waves: The Message

Grief waves can be sneaky. They are not always tied to specific memories or stimuli, and they may not always be obvious or even conscious. They can be more like the quiet rumbling of an idling engine. Cast your mind back to the last time you were going about your day and experienced a swell of grief. Before jumping into the story of *why* this happened, try to recall to the immediate sensation. Maybe a lump began to form in your throat, making it difficult to swallow. Maybe your eyes began to sting and you glanced upward to keep fresh tears from spilling. Maybe it even felt as though your heart leapt from its position in your chest. Now, bring yourself even further back to the moments and hours before. If you had listened very closely, could you have heard the rumbling? Maybe you could have and maybe not. Try to hear it right now. If the rumbling could talk, what would it say? Perhaps it would say, *You have been trying to hold it together for so long now* or, *You are more connected to this loss than you think,* or something else entirely. If you are open to it, take a few moments to explore this in a journal entry.

One way you can view your grief waves, particularly if they are feeling difficult to understand, is to consider them as invitations for you to meet a need. They may be signaling that there is something you did not know you needed. Maybe you are overdue for a big, messy cry. Perhaps your body is calling out for a shift in energy via gentle yoga, ecstatic dance, or a trip to your nearest Rage Room—contained spaces for expressing pent up emotions that are offered in many communities. These grief waves may also be signaling a need you have consciously suppressed. For example, you may need to share about the person you lost in community. More often than not, my clients are the people in their families and social circles who deeply desire a sense of connection around their loss. Two challenges tend to come up here. One is that they may not bring up their loved one for fear of being judged or perceived as "not over" the loss. The other is that they actually *have* made attempts to engage others on the subject, only to be met with distancing and rejecting responses. Eventually, they stop trying to connect out of self-preservation. If a wave is pointing to a need to speak of your loss, you can try to meet it, perhaps by joining a support group. By meeting our needs amid the waves of grief, we gain greater confidence in our ability to move through them.

Riding the Waves

It is helpful to accept the experience of grief waves as unavoidable. Further, consider that grief is not our enemy, but a sign of deep love and an unbroken bond with our person who died. Though much reflection can be done around these waves, you may be wondering what to do in the very moment they strike.

If it happens while you are out in public, try to find a quiet or private space, like the restroom or breakroom at work. Engage in simple box breathing, letting air enter your lungs slowly for a count of 4, holding for 4 seconds, and exhaling for 4 seconds. If it feels too overwhelming to hold the numbers in your mind, let them go. Check in with yourself and decide if you need to leave. If you are already home, prioritize your comfort to whatever extent you are able for the rest of the day or evening. When the storm begins to pass, you can start to reflect and process. I am going to guide you through an exercise you can use again and again, whenever a grief wave strikes, specifically tailored to you.

Grief Wave Plan

You can create a plan for grief waves that serves as a living, breathing document. You can fill it out and edit it over time, as you experience varying grief waves in your day-to-day life. A full planning document is available for download at http://www.newharbinger.com/55787. The purpose of the plan, inspired by the Safety Planning Intervention Tool (SPI), is to offer support in difficult moments (Stanley and Brown 2012). It is a resource to turn to for clarity about what you are feeling and what you need, as well as how you are going to realistically meet your needs. Its primary goal is to help you become compassionately curious about what will help you as you ride the waves of grief. Before creating your plan, think back to some of the waves you have experienced and consider the following:

- Where was I?

- Did anything in particular bring it on?

- How did I feel?

- What did I need?

- How did I cope with it?

With these reflections in mind, use a journal to record your answers to the following prompts, forming your very own Grief Wave Plan.

Grief Wave Triggers: What places, thoughts, images, and situations tend to bring up a wave of grief?

Grief Wave Warning Signs: What sorts of thoughts and emotions come up and signal a grief wave? How do they manifest in my body?

What I Need to Do During a Grief Wave: Do I need to cry? Or take a day off? Do I need time alone or time with others?

My Independent Grief Wave Coping Strategies: How can I bring myself comfort through the wave?

Someone Who Can Offer Extra Support: Who can I reach out to? How might I want them to support me through the wave?

Refer to this plan for helpful reminders the next time you find yourself in a wave. Keep in mind that the purpose of this resource is not to avoid a grief wave or stifle your emotions. It is merely an exercise in self-understanding, aimed at helping you carry yourself through a wave. The more you engage with them, the better you will be able to ride them.

Milestone Prompts

Here are a few questions to write about in your journal at some point ahead of your milestone event. If possible, set aside some time (at least thirty minutes to an hour) in a quiet, private space. Between work, caregiving, or both, setting time aside may be a feat in and of itself. If you have a trusted person in your life, who can in any way help grant you a pause from daily tasks, ask them for that help. My wish is that you will take this, your grief and your wellbeing, seriously—and that this trusted person will follow your cue. Continue to let this journey matter, even if your needs are not always understood. Settle into your space, close your eyes, and take some deep breaths to ground yourself. Then write responses to the following questions. Many emotions may arise, and this is okay.

- What milestone am I currently approaching?

- What am I feeling as this event draws closer?

- What would I share about this milestone with the person I am grieving?

- What might I need as I contend with my person's absence on this day? What about right before the milestone? What about right after?

- How can I carry them with me during my transition or celebration?

As you prepare for what may be a year's highlight or an event that turns the course of your life, know that your feelings and needs may shift and change. Check in with yourself and if needed, return to these questions to reconsider them.

Final Thoughts

Riding the waves of grief is part of how we integrate it into our lives. We accept its cyclical nature, its ebb and flow. Maybe grief "wave" even sounds too tame. As energy passes through ocean water, waves can softly lap at the shore's edge. When grief swells, it sends emotional winds whipping around us and it can shake the foundation beneath our feet. Perhaps "storm" is a better word. My father wanted that song from *Carousel* (and apparently, Liverpool FC) to carry me throughout my life without him and it has. Know that, when you are in the stormy part of grief, you are in some sense tapped into a community of people all over the world who live with loss. In that sense, you never will walk alone.

REFLECTION QUESTION

What do you know about your grief waves?

CHAPTER 6

Navigating a Changing Social Sphere

I have almost no recollection of anything my therapist said to me during the three years I worked with her after the death of my mother. As a therapist now myself, I can't recall any specific interventions or techniques she used, though I would have language for them now. And it doesn't matter. What I do remember is an instance in which I shared how much pain I was in, treading the water of a bottomless sorrow, frustrated by my perception that, at school, the loss seemed "over." During one session, her eyes misted over, filled with a layer of tears. She didn't sob or redirect the attention away from me—it wasn't therapeutically inappropriate. It was just what I needed. She silently communicated to me that she understood just how *bad* this was. I felt validated, vindicated even. *Yes, it makes sense that I feel this way.* Now, a different client may have needed something else in this moment, but when it comes to grief support, we mostly need to be seen and so often, we are not. This is where many relationships break down on the other side of loss.

Navigating our social world is a major component of how we integrate and grow through grief. We fear how it will look to others if they discover we are "still" grieving beyond a year or two or three or five or ten. Grief is both deeply individual and very, very social. When we are grieving a loss, our existing relationships change and, in some cases, they suffer. This is a subject that often causes tensions to flare. Notice any sensations you may be experiencing in your body already. Note that this chapter, in particular, may be beneficial for your loved ones to read as well.

Relationships on Shaky Ground

As we navigate the long-term integration of grief, it's common to experience instability in existing relationships. Relationship dynamics are unique—this is what makes them so life-enriching—so it is not possible to describe every variation of relational breakdown after loss. Still, what seems to most often cause friction between two people, whether one or both are grieving, is the sense of being misunderstood. After loss, we may become aware of the people in our lives who *get it,* the ones who don't get it but own that and show up anyway, the ones who don't get it and don't own that so they elbow in unceremoniously, and the ones who don't show up at all.

Silence

All too often, there is a code of silence around death and dying that extends to grief. As time goes on, we notice a drop-off in support. Then one day (for some this comes sooner than for others) it occurs to us that people in our lives do not address the loss, check in on us, or even mention our person. It is difficult to make sense of this. Of course, a knee-jerk reaction might be to think, *They just don't care.* Though only you know your relationships, consider that there are reasons this silence occurs that do not necessarily boil down to callousness. Still, these reasons make silence no less hurtful.

There are nuances to hold here. Many people have been fed the idea that the goal of healing in grief is to "move on." So their support involves not bringing it up. Likewise, if it has been a long time since the loss occurred, they may worry that mentioning it will upset us and "set us back" from some mystical, neat trajectory of healing. For some, it takes landing on the other side to realize this is a fallacy. Ultimately, people can't fully understand what they haven't lived, but this is where empathy must come into play.

Carl Rogers, a psychologist and the founder of person-centered therapy, provided a thorough definition of *empathy*. At its core, empathy is a process by which we "enter another's world without prejudice" (Rogers 1975). By setting aside preconceptions, taking the time to fully listen, and stepping inside our voiced experience of grief, they would know that our goal is not to cut ourselves off from the love we have for our person who died. Instead, we hope to learn how to carry this love and to exist in a new life—and new us—that has been shaped by this loss. This is something we may need to communicate to others, when we have the capacity.

Some people in our lives may feel distressed that they can't do anything to "fix" our grief. They may attempt to alleviate their sense of helplessness by telling themselves that we are probably "better." This relieves them from the imagined burden of having to gain magical powers to change our feelings. What we can tell them is that supporting us, in our grief, involves recognizing that they cannot change what has happened or what we feel—and that there is no need to change our feelings, even if it were possible. Instead, we need someone to enter our world, as Carl Rogers suggested. We need them to receive, hear, and see us, to meet us in the space between ignoring and fixing. This is where healing happens. It is also where relationships are saved from slipping through the cracks that loss hammers in the ground between people. When people don't communicate or practice empathy, assumptions are hatched and sometimes they are voiced aloud. People are not always silent and, in some moments, frustratedly, we may even wish they were.

Platitudes

Nothing communicates a lack of understanding to grieving people more than platitudes. These are some of the most common ones offered to the grieving:

- "Be strong."

- "At least...."

- "Time heals all wounds."

- "They're in a better place."

- "They're not in pain anymore."

- "They would want you to be happy."

- "We are never given more than we can handle."

- "Everything happens for a reason."

When you read from this list, what do you notice? Does one phrase stand out or sound familiar? What do you feel when you read it? *Platitudes* are phrases that have the appearance of being thoughtful but are overused and lack depth. People who attempt to fix usually barge in, with platitudes offered like Band-Aids to someone who needs a tourniquet. However, some of the phrases you read may not be offensive to you and you might even be comforted by them depending on your beliefs, worldview, and experiences.

The problem with platitudes is that they come with assumptions and can feel impersonal. It can be helpful for us and our relationships to keep in mind what might be behind them: people may fear straying from the beaten path of how society tells them to offer verbal support to the bereaved. Folks hear these phrases enough that they become introjected, subconsciously deemed acceptable and safe. They don't explore what platitudes actually mean until loss happens to them. The great irony of platitudes is that when speaking to grieving people like us, others may feel nervous, want to be gentle with us, fear "getting it wrong," and so they rely on these safe phrases—which come across as hollow. Thereby, they actually do in some ways "get it wrong." Sometimes people also name their own losses, but those losses differ in several facets (person who died, when, how, and so on), when attempting to lend verbal support. Though they are trying to connect, it can create comparisons when our raw grief should be the focus.

What might feel most helpful is to hear our people speak from their hearts with imperfect but deeply felt words: *This is so unfair for you to go through. I'm so sorry. I love you.* Or even, *I have no idea what to say. There aren't any words that would do this justice.* Try simply sharing with your loved ones that you don't actually need a solution—just their presence. To help you, I have written a Guide for Friends and Loved Ones that you can download online at http://www.newharbinger. com/55787 and give to others.

Anger

In response to feeling that our grief is misunderstood, we may feel angry in our relationships. I have often witnessed grieving people catch themselves in their frustration with others, wishing they understood why their words or behaviors are insensitive, and say, "Of course I don't want them to go through a loss like this." It is an understandable wish that people could somehow have the knowledge without experiencing the pain.

Just after my mother died, I learned that a group of friends went to the guidance office at school to discuss what had happened to me.

While I now see their bid for support in learning how to support me from a compassionate, matured lens, at the time I was resentful that they felt they needed someone to talk to. I thought: *But this is happening to* me, *not them. They get to go home today to their mothers.* How interesting that I even had any space left inside me to focus on this. Here is a distinction to make about anger: People will behave in ways we find odd and exasperating, and sometimes our anger is warranted. Yet sometimes...it is easier to direct anger toward living people, who we can have active conflict with, rather than feel our anger toward the death that took our person. This is ours to parse.

Pause and take a moment to notice how, if at all, anger has come up for you in your relationships. The next time it does, ask yourself, *What am I really angry about here?* If it truly is about something another has said or done, remind yourself, *If I value this relationship, I will address it.* This is how we can take care to not project anger onto loved ones who may not deserve it *and also* start meaningful dialogues where needed.

Envy

When we notice a distinction between others and ourselves, that we are now on the other side of loss where it has happened, while for them loss is still only a possibility, we may also feel envy. It is natural to have lost a loved one and then see someone in a similar relationship (like a marriage, friendship, or parent-child bond) and feel struck by the pain of wanting what they still have. It is not as though we want them to lack this relationship. It is merely a reminder of our loss.

When is the last time you felt like this? Being aware of your particular triggers and even writing them down can be helpful. You probably won't always be able to avoid the people who trigger your envy, as this would likely mean cutting yourself off from the world. But you can support yourself with compassionate mindfulness in the moment. It can help to observe, *This is really triggering my envy right now and that's okay.* We may also feel envious about a sense of innocence we perceive in others, an attitude toward life in which death happens else-where and time with loved ones is infinite. We might become stuck on this perception when we are feeling depressed and having difficulty connecting with hope. I will speak more about this in the next chapter.

Loneliness

We presumably gravitated toward the people in our lives, in part, because we shared some common ground. Grief can make it feel challenging to relate to your people one-on-one or to feel part of a social group, especially when you are the only one who has gone through a life-altering loss. When my parent-loss group for young adults comes together, members are often the only ones in their groups of friends who have lost a parent, given their age. Experiences like this create a fundamental feeling of being isolated and different from our peers. It is possible to feel lonely even while in the presence of others.

Secondary Loss

Not feeling understood in our grief, or anticipating that we won't be understood, typically leads to one of two outcomes. Believing that we won't get our emotional needs met, we distance ourselves, sometimes even becoming hyper-independent. Alternatively, our relationships may become high conflict, filled with emotional reactivity and frequent arguments that escalate quickly. What dictates this is a combination of various factors including personality, communication style, and the preexisting dynamics or unspoken "rules" of the relationship. When we don't share what we need, we thwart the opportunity to receive it and create room for resentment to grow like a third party in the relationship. Not addressing the feelings and obvious changes that are coming up can drive a wedge in friendships, marriages, and any kind of bond, placing them at risk of becoming secondary losses.

Repairing Inside and Coping Outside

We can do something about all this. Now, this may be a place where anger comes up, as you may think, *Why should I have to?!* You don't have to. Still, while it is important for others to educate themselves on grief, it may be helpful to remember the agency you possess in the co-creation and maintenance of your relationships. Notice what comes up as you read this next section.

Repair

To be very clear, I am not speaking about maintaining a relationship with someone who has been abusive. This is about relationships with human errors, communication breakdowns, hurts, yes, but not cruelties. It is vital to be discerning about the people we share our story with. Also, consider how clear you have been about what you need. I encourage you to maintain the self-respect to remember what you deserve and determine when to step away. There may be people we need to part with and grieve, and that is okay. However, having some continuity amid a major life upheaval helps us stay grounded. When someone has been historically safe, first try to talk to them about what is going on. This might mean sharing some of the grief and the changes you are noticing within yourself and the relationship. Notice what, if anything, feels immediately challenging about this. For some, it is the idea of being a "burden" to others. In the therapy room, inner-child and family-of-origin work can offer support for better understanding and deconstructing this fear. Yes, it can be frustrating, scary, and vulnerable to take on this conversation. But you may decide that it is worth it.

Here is an example of how to share what you need in order to avoid resentment, address your feelings, and protect your friendships. Let's say they utter a platitude. Take a moment to ground yourself and breathe. Check in with what you know about this person and your relationship. Calmly share that while you believe they are trying to be helpful, that isn't how their statement lands for you and you need something different. Focus on statements with "I" stems like, "I feel" or "I need," rather than "You are" or "You did." You might say something like, "Everyone experiences grief differently. Some people may find that statement helpful but personally, I don't feel comforted by the notion that my loved one would want me to be happy. Instead, it helps me to remember that they would accept any feelings that I have about their death."

Coping Outside

As we grapple with deciding where we want to repair our relationships, we also look to cope outside of them. This can mean forging new bonds or seeking solace in therapeutic settings. You may look into writing workshops, book clubs, or nonprofits designed to bring grieving people together. Though grieving people may find each other organically, groups are a very popular modality for grief therapy. They provide a container for members to hear about others' experiences, consider familiar feelings from new perspectives, learn new coping strategies, and share and be witnessed. When a group concludes after several weeks, the most consistent feedback that arises is relief and affirmation from having been seen. This is why grievers need to find each other and why talking about grief is healing in action. It is how we throw a lifeline to one another. Even individual therapy, when practiced relationally (hint: seek out a therapist who uses the term "relational therapy" in their profile) can be healing. The following list offers potential benefits to keep in mind. Make a note about what sounds most helpful and consider sharing this with a prospective therapist.

- Your therapist can act as a sounding board, as they are skilled in empathic, active listening.

- You can experiment with coping strategies that are tailored to you, rather than being pushed unsolicited advice.

- You can have space to fall apart and not censor yourself or "be strong" for the person in front of you, as the therapist is outside your circle and, while moved, they are unimpacted by the loss.

Grieving Alongside Family

Frequently, family members are not willing to grieve together. If you were already close with your family, this may have been the first place you looked for connection after loss. It can feel deeply upsetting and disturbing to discover that this is not always possible, at least how we think it should be. When two or more people are grieving a shared loss, there is still room for misunderstanding—each having their own ways of coping or not coping, their own relationships (to each other and the person who died), and their own familial roles. Sometimes, family members struggle to support each other because they are tending to their own grief. This is an all-too-common pain point for those who have lost a sibling. At the same time that you lost a sibling, your mother lost a child, and grappling with this may make it challenging for her to support you as she has in past hard times. We might hear platitudes less often within our immediate circles, but the silence can be just as unnerving. In some families, the person is remembered aloud and there might be a push to "remember the good times," while the grief isn't discussed. In others, the grief is touched upon but the person isn't discussed—it's too painful to remember how good they were. In both cases, there's discomfort being with difficult emotions.

I invite you to consider if this is something you would like to voice. By making yourself available to share grief together, you will have opened a door. While you leave it open, you do not need to wait to also seek support elsewhere. Many who join therapy groups are the sole members of their respective families willing to name the pain the whole family is experiencing. You may find that, with time, there are topics that your family members are willing to talk about and topics that feel precarious, for instance when a living parent begins to date. This may be a subject you bring to a group for outside support.

It can feel like a delicate act to determine where and when to repair and how to get our needs met. Ultimately, it may sound like a lot of work that we might not have the space for. Remember, every suggestion is an invitation. If you feel overwhelmed, return to this: the point is to be in connection, however that may happen. There may be further grief as we move out of connection with some people. As we move toward others, there may be big sighs of relief, morbid laughter, and despite not requesting admission, a gentle welcome into a club.

The Fear of Further Loss

Navigating relationships after loss is not just about smoothing out friction. We may also begin to fear further loss, relationally and literally. Once someone we love dies, loss becomes real and tangible. We are let in on the reality of the biggest open secret—that everyone really does die, even the people we see, hear, and touch on a daily basis. They are not exempt just because they are ours. It is terrifying to realize that it could, and one day will, happen again. One response to this fear is to distance ourselves from others and insulate from the impact of potential loss. This is a reactive adaptation to grief, a coping strategy, and it makes sense, but it is to our detriment. It heightens our loneliness and causes us to miss out on valuable connections and experiences that make life feel worth living despite the void of loss (Eisma et al. 2020).

You might also notice that the hypervigilance discussed earlier has not subsided. It can stick around and urge us to do things like call our partner or friend after we just saw them, to double check that they are okay. When we don't get an immediate response, fear whispers in our ear that the worst thing has happened. It holds us hostage until we receive a confused return call asking, *What's up?*, and we can finally breathe again. We can exhaust ourselves this way. In either case, we are working to gain control over what happens next because we are desperate to not have the rug pulled from beneath us again. We can't actually predict the future, as much as we want to. I know this may be difficult to read. It is a practice, at first perhaps a daily one, to acknowledge this and remind ourselves that we are in the present moment, not back there when the loss happened. Find a mantra to self-soothe with, such as: *I am safe. My people are safe. In this moment, we are okay.*

So much of the work before us is about making space for ourselves in the in-betweens. Distancing and clinging are not the only choices. We can cope by practicing staying present and leaning into our people, and we often do. We burrow into a shelter that is not promised to stand forever, even though we know it comes with emotional risk. To lose someone and then continue to stay soft and open to loving more people, equally as mortal, while deeply knowing the cost is an act of bravery that often goes unnoticed. And one that is worth celebrating.

Navigating a New Social Sphere

What about going to parties? Socializing with acquaintances in the outer layer of the friendsphere? Dating? Returning to the social world at large can feel like navigating new and unfamiliar terrain. Here are some ideas for reentry.

The Fear of Making it Awkward

At some point after loss, we interact with people we haven't seen since before the loss and with people who don't know what has taken place at all. We might wonder how we are going to address the elephant in the room, or if they don't know, when and how we are going to make them aware there's an elephant staring at us over their shoulder. The topic can become difficult to dodge. Why are we avoiding it? Their not-knowing may briefly suspend our reality, granting us some reprieve. We might also worry that we'll make things awkward by injecting seriousness into the conversation. In this way, even as grievers, we join others in the aforementioned code of silence or subtly alter the way we talk about it. For instance, when someone learns of the loss and says they're sorry, how do you usually respond? You may even have said, "It's okay." Really, what we are doing is attempting to protect their feelings. If this resonates, ask yourself: *Where did I learn this?* It might predate the loss.

When it comes to deciding when and how you tell people that a significant person in your life has died, whether recently or long ago, there is no right or wrong. Experiment with it. See what happens organically and follow what feels natural in the moment. Try different approaches and notice how you feel after. This does involve some risk-taking and, yes, there may be some awkwardness. But here's the thing: we went through the loss and if we can handle living with it, they can probably handle knowing about it. Talking about grief isn't a sign of pathology nor attention-seeking. It is not the downer we assume it must come across as. It is one way that we own our humanity and perhaps even inspire others to own theirs as well.

Making a Plan

If you have ventured to few social events and feel alarmed by the idea of relying on your intuition, there is something else you can try. Make a plan. A full version of the Socializing While Grieving Planner is available to download at http://www.newharbinger.com/55787. In brief, the plan can include:

- Where you're going, without any surprise pitstops

- How long you plan to stay (you can always stay longer)

- A tagline for responding about the grief, particularly if you are bracing for platitudes and pity, or don't feel ready nor open to having real conversations about the loss

- An identified support person

- A potential escape route

You may not need to write out a plan, although if you struggle to set boundaries this may serve as a helpful reminder for what you are and aren't willing to do. You might also benefit from making a plan if the loss is very fresh and socializing still feels new, it's been a while since you saw this group of people, the crowd is entirely new, or the event could be triggering. For example, you might plan to quietly slip away to the bathroom during the father-daughter dance at a wedding. You don't have to traverse these uncharted social waters alone. Consider the relationships that have remained close or have been strengthened through loss. Ask a friend to be "on call" to potentially exit with you. Ultimately, you may not need this. We can't predict how we will feel or control what happens. But we can form a guide to make it all feel a little less overwhelming.

Acknowledging Limited Capacity

In this chapter, I have mostly spoken about the challenges we face to get our needs met after loss. We might also notice the challenge of showing up how we want to. Relationships are a two-way street and we may feel guilt over our limited capacity to engage with others. We might feel we are not the friend we used to be. Noticing this is not all bad. It might be a helpful check-in. Consider where you would benefit from realistically adjusting your expectations for yourself, for the time being. Continually communicating this can help: "I haven't been feeling like myself since this happened. Thank you for being patient with me."

Final Thoughts

Grief challenges our relationships, and we will need to discern the ones worth saving. To do so, vulnerability is needed as supporters ask to enter the grieving person's world *and* grievers allow them entry. We benefit from forging new connections with other grievers too. While we may be able to share parts of our grief with others who haven't experienced life-altering loss, it is extremely validating to cultivate friendships with people who share the deeper layers of our experience. Relationships are not doomed because of grief. They may actually grow closer, which we'll explore soon. Next, let's consider the relationship you have with yourself. It is often this one that requires the most nurturing and discovery.

REFLECTION QUESTION

What do you most want the people in your life to know about your grief?

CHAPTER 7

A New Self

When Afton first sits down on the dark blue couch for her therapy session, she states some common opening lines: "So, this week, let me think. Things are okay." Then she pauses, glancing skeptically at the ceiling—like the words don't feel quite right. She shrugs before following up with, "I guess."

I gently query her, and with curiosity we wade through what it even means for things to be "okay," given the circumstances. Afton is thirty-five. Her cousin and best friend, five years younger than her, died a year ago. The loss is only just beginning to feel real, and that real feeling is bleak and scary. She recounts a family party over the weekend, where she fears that her cousin's absence might not have been on others' minds. Or that they were possibly trying to be brave for each other because the loss is just too awful, too tragic, to even name.

Typically, at past family parties, Afton and her cousin were in the corner, cracking long held, inside jokes. This shared language now feels as though it has evaporated, along with any words, really, even for the most mundane conversations. Afton wonders whether others noticed that she was withdrawn. The empty space where her cousin should be had been enlarged at a gathering of so many familiar faces, which didn't feel so familiar at all anymore. Everything felt foreign.

"Actually, I just don't feel like myself." Her eyes mist and I realize our conversation has hit something tender. She continues, "It's almost like, maybe, I don't even know how to be me without her."

As the session comes to a close, we are, together, somewhere far different from the place we started forty minutes ago.

Who Are We Without Them?

"I don't know how to be me without them."

"I don't know who I am anymore."

"I don't feel like myself yet."

These are phrases I hear often in the therapeutic space and you may recognize them in your own thoughts or conversations. There are some scary realizations to sit with in grief. One occurs when we stare at the expanse of time ahead and recognize, *Wow, I really have to live with this forever.* Another is when we begin to acknowledge a changed self. It's among the scariest realizations to sit with. Sometimes, depending on the phrasing, we may speak of expectations that—while unique— often reflect a sense of waiting to return to ourselves. Believing that we are going to find our old selves again after loss compounds our suffering. When we make this the goal, we become disoriented— similar to seeing ourselves in a funhouse mirror.

Please know: You are not lost, you are changing. While it's likely that you are not going to revert to exactly the person you were before loss, this doesn't mean that you are unfindable. Ultimately, you have an opportunity to forge a new identity, to be an active participant in this shift. But this does not need to be your goal right now. In this moment, all I ask is that you become curious. Here are some questions to begin reflecting on as you move through this chapter:

- Who do you feel you were before the loss?

- How would you have described yourself?

- How would others?

- Since the loss, how do you view yourself?

- How do you imagine others see you now?

You may want to write these questions down in a journal and write some brief responses—anything that first comes to mind. Notice how you describe yourself, particularly, before the loss. Does *parent, grandparent, child, grandchild, partner, sibling, caregiver, aunt, uncle, niece, nephew, cousin, friend* come up? (Please note, you are still that, always.) Many people explain who they are by stating who they are to others. This is intimately connected to feeling lost in grief.

How We See Ourselves

Why do we feel unlike ourselves after loss? Much of this has to do with the way that we saw ourselves in the first place. Our relationships and our life roles tend to shape our sense of self and sometimes the line between ourselves and another can become blurry.

Relationships and Life Roles

When we're asked "Who are you?", we tend to respond with identifiers like "I'm a wife, a caregiver, a teacher." We often define ourselves by our connections with others and see ourselves reflected back through the lenses of the various roles we play. After loss, the "Who are you?"

question becomes much more difficult to answer. If you feel alone in this or notice any self-judgments arising, know that this is natural. We have a helpful backdrop for understanding this in the form of the *self-expansion model*, developed by Arthur and Elaine Aron (1992).

According to this model, people incorporate loved ones into their own sense of self in order to enhance their self-efficacy and achievement of goals. This is thought to be largely positive. But when one of the two people in that relationship dies, it can be very disrupting and uprooting. We can feel like part of us, maybe even a lot of us, has gone with them.

You can visualize this model by imagining a pair of circles. Close your eyes and call to mind this image: you as one circle and your loved one as another. Do they overlap? By how much? The circles can be separated but close, cross over each other to varying extents, and even be totally merged. If the circles are very merged, you may find it particularly challenging to tap into a sense of your own self on the other side of loss.

The Line Between You and Another

Although common, identity challenges may or may not be a significant facet of your grief. After all, grief is universal and also unique for each of us. How much your sense of identity intersects with your grief, as well as how intensely you feel this effect, can be understood by considering two factors: self-concept clarity and event centrality. *Self-concept clarity* is essentially in the name. It means having a clear and steady view of your self. *Event-centrality* is your perception of how central an adverse event, like the death of a loved one, is to your life story or knowledge of who you are.

Research has found that when grieving people have reduced self-clarity, they experience higher symptom levels of depression and post-traumatic stress disorder (PTSD). These conclusions have concurred with prior findings that, if loss feels more central to self-identity, the griever experiences more pervasive distress (Boelen 2017). Check in with yourself about these concepts. How do they land within your experience? Perhaps this is why it has been so hard to see yourself after loss.

Here is an example of how these ideas can be lived out. If you were a caregiver for someone with a long-term illness and providing that care became the focal point of your daily life, you may have become disconnected from other parts of yourself. Without the role of caregiver, your self-concept today may feel unclear. This might be exacerbated if the loss of this person has felt central in your life. I want to let you know that it is okay to feel like the loss is a big part of your life and who you are now. You are not alone in this. The very fact that I am writing this book shows that, regardless of how many years pass, the loss of my parents has remained a core part of me. At the same time, I make space for other parts of me to emerge so that loss, while stitched into the fabric of who I am, does not consume my identity. I suspect that there is more to you than grief, even if anything else feels far out of reach right now.

Reactive Adaptation

As we try to live with loss, we might shift the ways we think about and interact with the world. Some of this change is conscious but much of it is unconscious. This is *reactive adaptation,* and everyone experiences it in some fashion. While we do this to achieve safety, we may sometimes unwittingly cause ourselves further pain in the process.

Reactive adaptation is essentially living in reaction to the pain of loss in ways that shape our lives around that anguish. This will look somewhat different for each person. As you read the following descriptions of how reactive adaptation occurs, consider the ways your beliefs and behaviors have been shifting as you grapple with your lived reality, as well as which emotions have taken center stage.

A Pessimistic Outlook

We might notice a sort of innocence in others who have not yet been through loss and become stuck, focusing on this when feeling depressed. In this clouded space, we are grasping at straws to understand what it means to be *us* without *them*, and our beliefs are at risk of shifting in a deleterious way. We might begin to hold a negative outlook, our thoughts becoming more black and white. We might think: *I have bad luck. If a bad thing is going to happen to anyone, it will probably be me. The odds are against me. Good things aren't meant for me.* Check in with yourself. Do any of these phrases sound familiar? Was there a time that they might have? Notice how true or untrue they feel for you, in this moment, as these sentiments represent where you are now, or what you used to feel but no longer do. Remember that our feelings can shift, as can our perspective.

Anxiety

We might begin to live in this pessimistic space, from these beliefs, with a depressed outlook and even an anxious one. A common companion to grief, anxiety can manifest in numerous ways. One is fear of further loss, as previously discussed. There may be anxiety about the separation from your loved one—the most extreme one that exists—and all that entails. Loss can also form an acute awareness of our own mortality and fragility, as we may sense that we're up against the clock, ruminate about dying as our loved one did, or hold back from taking risks. Some people report that their preexisting anxiety skyrockets after grief. Others say they would not have identified themselves as anxious prior to loss, but certainly do now. Sometimes anxiety isn't so attached to any specific thoughts or beliefs, and shows up as a general unease.

Fears of all that could go wrong can become palpable when a little voice chimes in to say that it probably will. I'd like you to pause for a moment and do something that might seem strange or silly. Notice how that voice sounds, in your mind. Does it tremble with vulnerability and fear? Imagine the voice is coming from a child, maybe a younger version of you, or even a sweet, innocent animal. Consider what you can do for the being expressing this anxiety. Maybe you take them in your arms or tell them, *I don't know exactly what is going to happen, but we will always figure it out.* Now, if the voice sounds threatening or like a know-it-all, give that voice a name—I mean, a name you *really* dislike. When it nags at you, say, "Go away, _____!" See what it's like to dismiss that voice, even with a roll of your eyes, and notice if it loses any of its power. Consider this a practice, as it may not have its intended effect on the first try.

Avoidance

Anxiety can be a powerful director of our actions and one way we try to quell it is to avoid. This might include withdrawing from work and play and the people around us (Eisma et al. 2020). Sometimes we become disconnected from the things we previously enjoyed doing, even if they were cornerstones of our identities. This will sometimes occur if those were shared activities with the person who died. We think, *How can I do this without them?* The experience may not feel the same. To be clear, it is completely okay if you truly don't feel a connection to this activity anymore. The key here is to discern whether or not you are holding yourself back from returning to something you love out of fear. Then you can decide if you are willing to challenge yourself to try, to just see how it feels to do that thing. Until then, it's difficult to be sure and there remains a chance that doing that thing could help you feel a little more like yourself, albeit a new version.

Another way that we react to loss is experiencing a crisis of faith or spirituality. We might even fully reject prior beliefs, now that an event has occurred which seems to contradict them. It may feel as though those beliefs must shift to accommodate the reality of loss. You might even feel anger toward a higher power. This can mark a major internal change, as spirituality or religion can be a crucial component of our identity and community. It may feel scary to question the beliefs that once held you. If this speaks to you, know that reassessing beliefs, resulting in either a shift or a return, is a natural response. Moving away from your spiritual practice is not necessarily avoidance. Remember, it's a matter of discernment. Here, especially, I encourage you to take your time.

Why It Hurts

So, what is the big deal? We're anxious, we curl into ourselves, and maybe we need to do that for a while. However, the more we disengage from life itself, the more we suffer. No longer engaging in activities we once enjoyed may further disconnect us from our sense of self. This amount of change can feel frightening, as we wonder, *What is there to hold on to?* We really need ourselves as a resource in order to get through the sharp edges of grief. Living in reaction hurts if it remains unconscious. It's not a place to stay, just like that early survival mode from chapter 3 is not a place to stay.

How to Work with This

Everyone will experience some internal shifts, and they don't follow a formula. For example, you may have withdrawn from others, not out of anxious avoidance, but because you feel too depressed to do much of anything. Anxiety may present itself when there is an activating event. Or anxiety may not be part of your grief story at all. If you are someone who likes to do things "correctly," I congratulate you for making it this far in the book, as there is not any one "right" way to do any of this. I also would like to let you know that if you see yourself in some of these reactions to loss, this is not a failing. It is actually you being resourceful.

Reactive adaptations are essentially ways that we consciously or unconsciously change our behavior in an effort to self-protect and feel safe. Bear in mind that this self-protection from the reality of loss is limiting in its true helpfulness. It's a Band-Aid. If you are avoiding engagement in your life, you likely feel that much more untethered from yourself—loss is painful enough without this. And really, on the other side of reactive adaptation, great growth is available. While these behaviors may feel like they are defining you now, please remember that they are not permanently affixed to who you are. They just represent a process you are moving through in the evolution of your survival.

We work through this by becoming consciously aware, discerning where we lack control and where we actually have agency. As I have been sharing various ways that we change in reaction to loss, I wonder what has been coming up for you. What examples from your own life came to mind? Now, sit with those things and ask yourself how you feel about them. Maybe you feel okay about your spirituality being under review but distressed about the distance between yourself and others. Maybe you are nervous about questions you now have regarding your career choice. Maybe you resonate with anxiety about your own mortality, but when you step back, you feel able to cope with this as you live your day-to-day life.

Show yourself compassion in the form of affirmation. For example, "It makes sense that being close to others feels scary right now." Trade in judgment for curiosity. Ask yourself: *What feels safe for me about [insert reactive coping mechanism]? Can I notice and feel a part of me that wants to act differently?* I want you to know that as much as loss has taken from you, you do not have to live in reaction to it, if you don't want to. You don't have to contort your existence according to the shape of this pain. Things won't change overnight, but if you can be patient with yourself and take stock of what is and isn't working for you, you will already be on your way to growing through this.

Purposeful Growth

Not all changes after loss are a cause for concern. Loss can lead us to live reactively, but it can also inspire us to live with new intention. Even as it, of course, takes away a person, rhythms and routines, purpose, and confidence about our place in the world, it can also, somehow...give. If you feel incredulous about this, I understand. You might even want to shut the book. That's okay—you can come back at any time and go at your own pace. Just know that I'm not going to end this chapter by saying growth makes loss worth it or serves as a consolation prize. Of course, we'd give back all the wisdom just to have our person here. Maybe we can agree that loss has a lot of gray space and encourages us to live between binaries, to hold nuance. It's not that loss is a good thing. It's actually, dare I say it, the worst. Once it has happened, we can dig further into that, sitting in the abject awfulness of it, and really, we need to do some of that. However, it is very possible for loss to change us in such a way that we make conscious and intentional choices that improve our way of life. We couldn't control or prevent loss from happening. But now that it has, we can decide what we want to do with that reality, seeking peace and contentment, maybe even stretching our imaginations to reach for joy. Loss can *inform* how we move forward rather than *dictate* how we remain stuck.

Crystallized Values

Some growth after loss happens without conscious effort, but when we struggle with a hazy self-perception, it is helpful to intentionally foster personal values and goals in order to clarify that picture (Boelen 2017). My clients often tell me they notice a values shift—things that used to seem important no longer do and new things become the focus. For example, perhaps it was all about work before and now you really want to prioritize spending more time with loved ones. Maybe loss has softened your perspective on an old conflict or you no longer feel as reactive to petty disagreements. Loss can serve as this check-in point about what really, truly matters when all is said and done. We might feel released by this. Take a moment to consider any shifts in your values since your loss happened.

Attunement to Self

You may be like some of the people I have companioned through grief, new to therapy and doing the brave work of attuning to and naming emotions for the first time. Through this work of identifying and vocalizing your emotions, your relationships can benefit. Attunement to yourself may also grant respite from a need to perform, guiding you to release your grip on how others might perceive you. Being the most authentic version of who you are is a wonderful way to find your people.

Motivation to Truly Live

We can reframe the emptiness that grief brings as openness, like a canvas waiting for fresh paint. You don't have to be excited about it. What if you just thought to yourself, *What do I have to lose?* You may then want to act on this, exploring new possibilities—a new calling, career shift, maybe becoming involved with a meaningful cause. Proximity to death can bring about anxiety but it can also bring about positive activation. The very same recognition of just how fragile and short life is asks: *What do you want to do with life while you have it?* Rather than becoming frozen by that thought, we can mindfully move forward from it. You may have heard the term *posttraumatic growth*, which is essentially positive change after suffering. Two domains of this growth include an appreciation for life and an existential under-standing of self (Calhoun et al. 2010). Loss urges us to practice attun-ement to our emotions and desires, which can help us make more authentic choices as we move through this one existence.

A Strengthened Self

Another domain of posttraumatic growth is perceiving ourselves to be "more vulnerable, yet stronger" (Calhoun et al. 2010). Though we have sharper awareness of how vulnerable we are in this life, we might also come through loss knowing what we can weather. Here's a very simple example I see often: People have an aspect of their academic or work life that feels very challenging. What helps them get through when they are feeling anxious or even doomed is to remember what they have overcome. They think, *If I could survive life-altering loss, I can probably survive this project.* They remember that while loss can't be solved, other things in life can. We can come back to this insight when new challenges arise.

A New Connection

We can also grow through grief in the very connection we are longing for. Though we can't be with our person physically, we might be able to experience their presence differently. While your beliefs may be in question, you may consider exploring spirituality in a newfound or deepened way, tapping into an intuition about the afterlife that has always been there or maybe believing in it for the very first time. We can reach this person we love so much in a way that is immaterial yet somehow extremely close. We'll explore this further in chapters to come.

Meeting Complex Feelings

If all these words about growth feel unrealistic, you may not yet be in a place to receive them. They may not authentically match where you are. This is okay. You don't have to force them to feel real, and no one outside you can dictate when and how you grow. In fact, most of us have to go through living in response to the loss, sifting through all the confusion, before we can become ready for any purposeful growth. For now, return to noticing any changes in yourself.

When you notice that you have had the capacity to make meaningful changes in response to your grief, you might experience another feeling: guilt. When we recognize that we are moving out of survival into peace, we might feel as though we are betraying our loved one. We might think, *How could anything good possibly come of their death?* I encourage you to remember that growth after loss is a matter of *both/ and*: we can experience *both* deep gratitude for the wisdom we have gained in life *and* also make space for the sadness or anger we feel about what prompted such growth. Grief need not define you, and the resilience that grows from profound loss may become a part of you that is a source of pride.

Me, Before and After Loss Exercise

Perhaps you are now aware that something has shifted within you. As you take steps toward understanding and making peace with these specific changes, maybe you need some more clarity around them. The following exercise is intended to help anchor this work as you learn about this emerging version of yourself after loss.

This exercise is very simple and provides a lot of room for you to make it your own. You can do this completely freeform by drawing on a blank piece of paper or in a journal—or you can download a worksheet at http://www.newharbinger.com/55787 to print and complete. If you are not feeling ready to do the exercise, you can simply read on to understand its purpose.

Draw the outlines of two bodies or use the worksheet available online. Label one body outline "Me, before" and label the other "Me, after." Then write or draw any traits, emotions, physical sensations, or behaviors you have possessed, felt, or enacted—before and after loss.

Display them inside or outside the lines of the body, depending on whether or not you believe they are visible to others.

Notice what comes up for you in response to this image and prompt. Maybe you feel curiosity or apprehension and think, *I don't want to do this.* Take a pause to ground yourself. If you decide to continue, go at your own pace and try to be as uncensored as possible.

When you're done, look at what has changed between the two outlines. You might see a mix of reactive adaptations and hints of purposeful growth. You may notice that some parts of you have disappeared and others are totally new. How does this feel to see? Maybe scary or even validating?

Then notice what has remained the same, even if it's small. This is just as important to recognize, so you remember there are still stabilizing forces in your life. Perhaps you feel some relief about that. Overall, notice if there were any surprises for you.

Final Thoughts

Loss changes us because our identities are deeply informed by our closest connections. We may live in reaction to loss, just trying to stay safe. But there is growth available to us when we are willing to try parting with some of those safety strategies. Keep in mind that we often don't just experience either *reactivity* or *growth*. We might intermittently feel anxious or depressed, at other times feel inspired—even straddle it all—growing in some ways, reacting in others. You might wonder if you are "on track," but identity work usually does not happen immediately after a loss. This is deeper grief work, and in some ways, it is the work of a lifetime as we continue to evolve. Grief expert Elisabeth Kübler-Ross once said that "Beautiful people do not just happen" (1975). You might ask: *Just how much of me goes with them? How much remains? What if, in part, I get to decide?* In the next chapter, we will dive into how to take charge of the story.

REFLECTION QUESTION

What do you miss about your past self? What do you appreciate about yourself as you are now?

CHAPTER 8

Writing a New Story

To be honest with you, after my mother died and my position in this world as a parentless person was solidified, I felt that my life was over. To be *totally* honest with you, there were times I even felt apathetic about how my life turned out. I was hung up on the *why* of it all. Why was I born to these parents, only for them to shortly afterward leave the Earth where they brought me? I couldn't find an answer or a reason, so at some point I made a choice to paradoxically accept the *not knowing*.

Once I had more stable ground beneath me, having moved out of survival mode, I felt compelled to go and make a new reality for myself. I wanted to leave the rest behind, almost as if the losses hadn't happened, almost as if it wasn't real at all. It was too painful to be with. This lasted awhile, but eventually when grief proved unignorable, the thought of the love and the loss all being for nothing became excruciating. In some sense, I had to make it *for* something. Today, I might answer the question "What was all of this for?" by saying that the love my parents gave me is something I get to keep forever, and the loss of my parents deepens my desire to share that love. This is an example of how we make meaning of our loss, which I mentioned earlier in the book. It's something no one can give to us, and it actually feels repulsive when others try to push it on us with platitudes like, "God needed an angel." Meaning is something we only find through our own experience, sometimes when we're no longer looking.

Loss can feel like the end of our story—and it will be, if we let it. Or we can keep writing. By "writing," I mean that we can create a new story, or we might pick up the pen and continue as the new, changed-by-loss versions of ourselves. We can be intentional about how we walk through the world, choosing to move with the curve of the path. This matters. Our life stories are important—they are a core part of our identities because they are the vehicle through which we integrate our experiences (Thomsen et al. 2018). They help us make sense of how we have become who we are and understand where we would like to go.

Think back to any discoveries you made about yourself in the last chapter, even if it was just a couple of things, even if they feel small, even if you don't know much about them yet. I am going to offer you a framework for deciding what to do with these changes you have found. You can align them with action toward a life that, while irrevocably changed, also feels good. Maybe you have discovered that through loss, helping others feels important to you. You might translate this into action by getting involved in a nonprofit organization. Maybe you have discovered a newfound appreciation of the little things. You might consider waking up early to watch the sunrise and feel awe at it.

Let's address some feelings you may have coming into this chapter. The future is a scary prospect for the grieving. It's normal to feel lost and unable to picture a future because your person will no longer be in it. It might even feel like the best is behind you and there is little to look forward to. To start, rest assured that you do not need to create a roadmap for the rest of your life. All you need to do is take it day by day, remembering that we are not writing your person out of the story—we're simply helping you continue to live fully. There may also be days when you feel so angry or resentful about what has happened that the motivation to create some good for yourself just isn't there. We can't make every day a triumph or a beautiful tribute to our loved one. We have to be allowed to just be human and have really hard days. What I'm going to offer you here are simply further invitations.

Releasing, Reclaiming, and (Re)building

Perhaps at this point you have begun to reflect on changes in your beliefs, your emotional landscape, and your embodied experience of being in the world. You may have a better grasp on specific parts of yourself to look at—those that seem to have faded, those that seem to have remained, and those that seem new and unfamiliar. You might have strong feelings about these changes. Still, consider that they are likely to evolve, ebb, and flow as grief does—especially as you live more life, take on new roles, and encounter milestones. You might be wondering what to do with this information about yourself. First, see if you can return to some degree of radical acceptance by affirming yourself with something like this: *I am probably not going to return to exactly the person I was before loss. Without them here in my physical world, the day-to-day experience of my life is fundamentally different now. In some ways, so am I.* Remember, radical acceptance means acknowledgment—not approval—and it will be more or less challenging depending on the day, what is going on, and how much support you have. You can start to rework and realign your sense of identity and personal world by engaging in the Three Rs: Release, Reclaim, and (Re)build.

Release

Part of growing through grief means grieving more than just the person who died. It also means grieving parts of yourself, the life you lived with them, and the experiences you won't be able to have with them. This releasing is a practice in discerning what needs to stay and what needs to go, so that you are not weighed down by the dissonance between *what was* and *what is*. What do we decide to let go of? And how do we do it? Let's explore these questions.

WHAT WE RELEASE

We release the parts of self that feel truly gone. You may be able to identify these parts through reflection in your day-to-day life, through an individual or group therapy session, or even the *Me, Before and After Loss Exercise* in the last chapter. For example, you may no longer feel connected to your career and recognize the need for a change, as daunting as that may be. We might also release the armor we have developed in response to loss, like self-isolation. You may at some point realize that you are closing yourself off to new connections with others. As you come to understand that this is a way of living in reaction to the loss, you may make a conscious choice to begin letting that self-protective mechanism go by letting someone in.

Only you can determine what you need to let go and are willing to release after loss. It's not for anyone else to say. This is probably the most challenging part of forming a new path forward because why would you want to experience any more loss? You might not want to release something, but in order to care for yourself you recognize that it needs to go. I encourage you to find a gentle space to talk about this experience and decision.

HOW WE RELEASE IT

Releasing can include shifting your perception, but it can also be quite tangible. We may need to actively release through a mourning practice. Let's consider, for example, a man who has been a caregiver for his chronically ill uncle for his entire young adulthood, until this beloved family member died. He has little sense of himself outside of this role, though he was glad to take it on. A mourning practice for him might include gathering some objects related to his caregiving and creating a ceremony around parting with them. To be clear, I do not mean just throwing them in the garbage. It's important to spend time being with the feelings that the objects evoke and mindfully parting with them, perhaps choosing something to keep. This is mostly symbolic. Another example could include creating an altar that represents a part of yourself that you feel ready to say goodbye to, spending time at that altar, and then gently clearing it. Practices like these can be done in solitude or in community.

Pause to ask yourself: What might you need to release? How might you do so? When you engage in this practice, would you like to be on your own or in the company of someone else?

Reclaim

Some parts of yourself and life as you have known it will remain steady through grief. Maybe your humor has remained intact, although perhaps it has become a bit darker. Maybe your spiritual beliefs remain, although your connection to them has loosened as you haven't been as engaged. Check in about what parts may still be there for you.

WHAT WE RECLAIM

We look at these parts of ourselves that have, to some degree, remained. We reclaim those parts that we feel ready to lean into again. Maybe a constant for you has been feeling grounded in your yoga practice and finding solace there. You might more fully reclaim your practice by intentionally creating more time and space for it. In doing so, you may become more anchored in a familiar sense of self. We also reclaim elements of our identity and old life that feel recoverable, where we may have caught little glimpses of these facets of self coming back. For example, it could be grounding to realize that you have let out a deep belly laugh for the first time since the loss. Pause to notice the fact that your capacity to do so is returning. Laughter is something we really need—it's important for our survival to be able to reclaim that. None of this happens overnight, so as we reclaim, we must practice patience with ourselves. If you are working through this with a therapist or in a group, you would probably benefit from their patience as well and may want to communicate this.

HOW WE RECLAIM IT

The elements of identity that you may want to reclaim could be something as simple as reconnecting to your lightheartedness, to laughter. They could also be very closely linked with the loss itself. You may want to reclaim, or stay close to, your identity as a parent, a child, or a partner—in whatever capacity you now can. You can support this identity through ritual and social support. Research has shown that bereaved parents may negotiate their identities after the loss of a child by engaging in rituals such as tending to a memorial site alone or with loved ones. In a sense, they continue to parent while acknowledging deep grief (Toller 2008). A more recent study compiled interviews with bereaved spouses and found that the process of identity reconciliation was in part facilitated by social support. These supports can help you experience catharsis through talking about a spouse, validating a spouse's memory, and in some cases, reinforcing your sense of belonging in a family you may have joined through the relationship. Spouses can reclaim marital identity and bond with the departed by celebrating memories (Wehrman 2023).

Whatever you seek to reclaim, begin considering rituals you could create by tapping into when, where, with whom, and in what situations you feel most connected to that part of yourself.

(Re)Build

As you begin forming the next part of your life, there are likely newfound parts of yourself to build upon. You may have reclaimed something and wish to continue building it back up. Here, we foster hope for what could lie ahead.

WHAT WE (RE)BUILD

Bring yourself back to the *Me, Before and After Loss Exercise* from the last chapter. Look at the image of yourself after loss and notice what has newly appeared. Is there anything that feels at least mildly intriguing or maybe even exciting? Something that makes you feel proud of yourself? Something you'd like to explore further?

HOW WE (RE)BUILD IT

There is no rush to (re)build or experience any positive feelings associated with, or stemming from, your loss. It is okay to be where you are. Understandably, if someone were to overemphasize hope or overlook the depth of your pain in favor of focusing *solely* on growth, it might feel like they are pushing a "silver lining." Instead, consider striking a balance between honoring your loss and looking to the future, so you can put some good in it. Brainstorm some ways to embark upon self-discovery. For example, after your loss, you may feel compelled to be with others and support them. Perhaps you could get involved in some volunteer work and find purpose in this. Maybe you want to build upon social connections with other bereaved people.

In this way, we can begin forging a new sense of self and a new path forward in this life by releasing what no longer feels like ours to keep, reclaiming what so palpably does, and (re)building through a process of self-discovery. One example of how we can release, reclaim, and (re)build is intentionally navigating the holidays. Holidays are among the hardest parts of adapting to loss. There might be pressure around you to enjoy yourself (or you might feel guilt for doing so), to part with traditions (this may feel like too much change) or keep traditions that no longer feel right. If you have already experienced your first big holiday since the loss, take a moment to reflect. What parts of the experience felt impossible to recapture? What aspects felt steady and consistent, despite how much has changed? What new parts, if any, did you actually like? Use these reflections to consider how you may want to approach the holiday next year, keeping what feels right and making space for new rituals. To support you in practices like this one, there is a worksheet available for download at http://www.newharbinger.com/55787 that offers journaling prompts for each of the Three Rs. Take your time with them and consider sharing what you have found with a trusted support person.

Taking Charge of Our Story

Was that really me? Watching old home videos or looking at photos that include your person can be a surreal experience. How strange it might feel to compare that life and this life you're in now. They are one in the same, though they look so different. Despite the massive interruption of loss, the tidal wave of change, this life has actually been continuous. The thought may cross your mind, *These poor people don't know what's coming.* Subtly, the you that is on the screen becomes someone else. You may feel struck by seeing friends still doing activities with family that they did when they were kids, their lives seemingly full of continuity where yours may have a stark sense of *before* and *after* loss. There may be several closed chapters in your life, some traditions lost. Perhaps you feel as if a whole book came to an end and you became someone else, floating through space without anchors to remind you that *this is you and these are the things you do with your people.* You might wonder if people you meet after loss really know you. You also wonder if you really know you. Life with loss can feel like a life fragmented. It can feel like having lived many lives. It can feel like having been many people. Loss creates a sharp break in the continuity of our life story (Thomsen et al. 2018).

This is why releasing, reclaiming, and (re)building can be so impactful—it allows us to begin putting together a cohesive picture of ourselves and our lives. *Narrative identity* is something we form by making connections between our past and present. It is believed to help us understand our reactions to loss (Thomsen et al. 2018). We take stock of where and who we've been, where and who we are now, and take back enough of our power to say who and where we want to be. We are acknowledging that grief changes us and will remain because, in some ways, it lasts as long as the loss does. We're not bypassing that. And yet, a sense of wholeness within remains possible. It is also helpful to find small ways to look toward the future and feel good about what you envision.

Crafting a Positive Future Story

Loss makes the future unclear. A significant person, alive in our past and maybe even recent present, is no longer going to physically be part of chapters to come. You might have wondered what it will be like to celebrate the holidays, walk down the aisle, or even run errands without talking to them on the phone as you do it. It might be hard to feel that there is anything to look forward to if they are not going to be there. However, research supports that crafting a positive future life story is key for coping with grief (Thomsen et al. 2018). We don't have to think that it's all going to be smooth sailing, as much as we wish we had ticked the box on major loss and will therefore be relieved of any future ones. But can we believe that alongside future hardships, there will also be good?

Sure, we are working with the evidence that we have—loss does happen. Pause and notice if you can find some competing evidence, memories of bright spots in your life. When I ask if you can believe you'll experience bright spots again, notice what your gut says. It's okay if you are not yet in a place to say yes. Growing through grief happens when we honor all of our feelings, including our deep sadness as well as our hope. It takes practice to foster the latter.

Rather than speculating on whether or not there will be anything to look forward to, we might have to take the first step of creating it.

We can fill in the empty corners by making plans, whether big or small. Here is one way to begin. Create a list in your journal or on your phone of every moment you feel a little spark—even if it's the tiniest spark you've ever felt. Maybe your curiosity about a class is piqued, or you feel interested when you see an ad for a museum exhibit. Whenever they pop up, write these down. Try not to underestimate the power of curiosity, interest, and desire after how bleak and dull things may have felt in the beginning of your journey through loss. Pick something from the list and decide whether you want to do it alone or with someone else. In the case of the latter, talk about it with them. Put it on your calendar and notice over time how it feels to look forward. The goal isn't to mindlessly fill a calendar, but to create little events that spark something like joy. If you're more of a visual person, flip through magazines and cut out pictures that represent things you may want to do. Use these images to create a vision board.

Writing It into Existence

Another way to rebuild identity and the life story disrupted by loss is through expressive writing and the use of memoir (Den Elzen 2021). We can contain the *before* and *after* loss as separate chapters in one book, honoring what was and holding hope for what will be. You don't actually have to write a memoir, unless you feel called to. It can remain private and just be for you if that's what feels right. It can also be simple in structure and casual in practice. If school essays drained you of any desire to write or you often came away feeling that writing wasn't a strength, try not to underestimate yourself. But also don't pressure yourself to form strict assignments out of your grief. If you ever feel overwhelmed with thoughts about the big picture of your life, start writing, even short notes to yourself, and see what comes out. Consider these prompts if you need help getting started:

- In addition to my person, what else has loss taken from me? How important is it to me to get those things back?

- Since the loss, where have I been feeling most stuck?

- How has loss propelled me forward in new ways? If it hasn't, how would I like it to?

- Are there any changes that loss created in my life or within myself, whether negative or maybe even positive, that I feel curious about?

Reading memoirs on grief is considered particularly helpful for those who are widowed. It has been proposed that these memoirs could be used in therapy as a processing tool, though more research is needed (Den Elzen 2021). Regardless of the type of loss you have experienced, if you come across a memoir about grief that resonates for you, consider highlighting the passages that most speak to you and bringing them to therapy sessions.

There may be some parts of your story—particularly those that lead you to feel out of control—that you may wish to rewrite, not in the literal sense, but in how you walk through the world.

Rewriting Old Stories

We don't only write a new story by putting pen to paper. We write a new story metaphorically when we are intentional about the way we walk through the world, choosing to live a full life and not letting loss define what we get to experience. We also write a new story when we declare through action that loss, though instrumental in our lives, does not rule us. An example is your health. Like many, you may experience anxiety when going to a doctor's appointment, knowing it's likely you'll have to recount the family medical history tied to your loss. You may leave that appointment feeling deflated, thrown back into the rawness of early grief.

Cary recently turned twenty-six. No longer on his parent's insurance plan, he has been putting off his yearly physical with a new doctor, not just because it's another task on the to-do list, but because the thought of it brings up anxiety. Four years ago, Cary's older brother died from a hereditary condition and he anticipates that this loss will come up when his family medical history is taken. After rescheduling the appointment several times, Cary challenges himself to follow through. He practices grounding exercises the night before and on the way to the appointment. He later shares with me that, "I decided to just own it. This is part of my family medical history. I don't have control over it, but I am taking steps to manage my own health. I think I can feel proud of that."

Over time, Cary feels less discomfort uttering the words about his brother's illness and passing, largely because he can reframe what it means to state them. He could have opted for a lifetime of avoidance, succumbing to the fear of dying from that same illness. This would be understandable. However, he chose to write a story of empowerment around it. Consider a sensitive aspect of your loss that could lead you to shut down, withdraw, or avoid parts of life. What small action could you take to counteract this? What alternate story could you tell about it?

Meeting the Feelings

What has come up for you while reading this chapter? Hope? Fear? Anger? It is all welcome. It's completely natural to have a hard time believing that life will be good again. However, if you experience a complete lack of desire to continue on with life, I would strongly encourage you to seek further support.

SUICIDAL IDEATION

Though too often shrouded in stigma, *suicidal ideation (SI)* is something that can occur in the midst of grief. There is *passive SI* (like thoughts about not wanting to wake up) and there is *active SI* (thoughts about killing yourself). Often in grief, SI is linked to a desire to be with the person we have lost. It's important to have these thoughts assessed by a professional who is knowledgeable and compassionate. You don't have to sit with any of these thoughts alone. If you are experiencing thoughts about killing yourself, you can get help immediately by calling the 988 Lifeline.

Now you have some tools to consider, including: answering journal prompts, keeping a list of what sparks your interest, and reframing an aspect of loss in a way that feels empowering. You might feel curious to try these, but apprehensive about what will meet you on the other side. The very idea of a new story can feel daunting. So can trying new things, starting another career, moving, or entering into relationships with people who never knew our person. We might fear that this will make them feel further away. Will it all feel like a dream, that old life where they were here with us? If we sever the connection by suppressing our grief and our memories, it may feel this way. Given that you're reading this book, I suspect that won't be the way you move through this.

We return to choice. Are you willing to live in service of your fear and risk feeling further distance from yourself? True, there may be moments of sorrow when you realize what your person is missing, what they have missed. But is apprehension about continuing on worth never having new experiences, relationships, or enjoyment in this life you are still here to live? Continue to meet the feelings. But know there is a choice available to you to continue writing, even as you feel them. You don't need to reject those feelings. In fact, acknowledging them and making space for them is what might enable you to continue growing through this. The fear of leaving behind a loved one who has died is a common one, but you truly don't need to leave them behind at all in order to keep living.

Final Thoughts

Loss can be a meaningful, deeply impactful part of our story—yet it doesn't have to be the whole story. We can keep writing the story, one that honors the past and builds a bridge to the future. We can release, reclaim, and (re)build by reaching into the past and doing things that help us feel continuity in our lives. We can create new plans to look forward to enacting. As we engage in writing our story, we also take charge of our personal narratives out in the world. Loss is unreturnable, though we can choose to grow from it. However, please know that you do not always need to turn your pain into purpose. I believe that you can make good happen for yourself in this changed life. I also believe your grief matters on all the days when you can't make it into something beautiful and the pain is just pain. If the fear of moving forward continues to nag at you, know that as you write a new story, your loved one can be part of it. You can write them into the continuation of your story. Next, we'll consider how to do that.

REFLECTION QUESTIONS

How has loss changed the story of your life so far? How would you like to impact the story of your life going forward?

CHAPTER 9

Staying Connected

As the stories of our lives continue to unfold, and we intentionally practice continual surrender to all that has changed within and around us, we do adapt. We begin to breathe again, with an ease that once felt totally inaccessible. Yet, as time moves forward, we also experience the fuller effects of our loved one's absence. Your relationship with your person who died doesn't have to go away and it also doesn't have to remain stagnant. Contrary to outdated notions about how to continue on after loss, we actually do not need to disconnect from our loved ones when they die or leave them behind. In fact, keeping them close to us may become a key part of living a contented, fulfilled life. Just as we grow through our grief and our life path takes a new course, our relationship to the person who died also transforms. Of course, it is not the same as having them physically present with us. You have lost someone close to you in the physical world. Now, if you would like to maintain that closeness, you are tasked with finding ways to encounter them beyond the limits of time and space. Whether spiritual or not, it is natural to long for their presence. Either way, regardless of your beliefs, consider that it is very possible to maintain a connection with them.

A Pull to Connect

Sometimes, you may receive a reminder of your person and suddenly realize that you haven't consciously thought about them that day or that week. Perhaps you had become quite busy within your world, your new version of normal. They may feel further away than you have, somehow, become accustomed. This is where guilt may seep in. You might think, *How could I ever not think about them?* If this surfaces, remind yourself that this is a natural occurrence and may signify that you have actually been present in your day-to-day life—something likely helpful for your wellbeing.

Consider the reflexes we touched upon earlier, like the instinct to pick up the phone to call them. These may gradually transform into wishes. As we walk through the world for many months and years, learning to inhabit a life that they no longer occupy, we somehow, almost become used to their absence, as uncomfortable as this may feel to admit. Then one day, we receive amazing news and feel a swell of joy or pride and experience a reflexive urge to call the one person we can't. We feel suddenly very unused to it. It may feel like they were just here yesterday, the loss becoming fresh again. Yet it's as though we've lived a whole lifetime without them.

Many people experience a vague void-like sensation and curiosity before or on significant days. For example, on your birthday you may receive some messages from loved ones, carry out whatever plans you have, and at the end think, *Hmm, it feels like there's someone I didn't talk to today.* It takes a moment to dawn on you and then the loss falls on you, hard. In these moments, it's helpful to remember that you can still talk to them.

Connecting Spiritually

I am at the cemetery on a sunny spring day. It has been years since I last visited and I have no idea what I expect to feel. I crouch down to read the headstone, taking in their names and dates of life, taking in the reality of what happened to my family. Then I lie down on the cool green grass, as if attempting to inch my way just a little closer to them, and let my eyes close. The feeling of a warm, ethereal embrace wraps around me and though I am surprised by the intensity of this sensation, I welcome it. When my eyes flit open to the sky above, two birds fly past and immediately, without any question or analysis, I know it's them.

What I am describing is a sign. After loss, many people experience this phenomenon of receiving signs from loved ones who have moved on from this life. Some experience them shortly after loss or only years later, frequently or spread out over time. You can think of signs as a wave hello from the other side, a message that often seems to most simply say, *I'm here with you.* Words can't capture the clarity that washes over us when we receive that communication. It just is. If you are prone to over-intellectualizing, you may second-guess what you felt in that moment. But ultimately, when we know, we know. It is a felt sense. In some instances, our people transmit signs through symbols, objects, media, or elements of the natural world that are significant to the relationship. For example, they cross your mind as you go through your morning routine, then when you start the car you hear their favorite song on the radio. Signs can be channeled through less significant objects at the exact moment we are thinking of our person. One common example is lights flickering when we have just called them to mind or spoken about them. I had never related birds with my parents. But that day at the cemetery, I knew in my bones that they were greeting me this way.

Perhaps you have experienced a sign. Think back to a time when you felt as though you were not alone, despite being by yourself. Or recall a time when something too coincidental occurred. Notice what feelings come up as you conjure this memory and keep them in mind as you read on.

When we receive signs, we may feel immense comfort. Although these moments in no way compensate for their physical absence or make the loss acceptable to us, they can renew a sense of connection that brings some solace. Laura Lynne Jackson (2015) captures the essence of signs beautifully when she writes, "Grief brings us great pain, but the Other Side teaches us that this pain is not about the absence of love—it's about the continuation of that love." When the song comes on the radio or lights flicker or birds fly overhead, we can be soothed by the knowledge that our people are even infinitesimally closer to us than we believed them to be. Yet, many emotions come up around receiving, or even thinking about, signs and not all of them are warm and consoling.

A raw intensity can be provoked by this greeting, especially when we are not expecting or wishing for it. It can reopen some of the grief we keep zipped up when we are out in the world. If you attend a medium reading, where a psychic medium acts as a conduit between you and your loved one, you may have a similar emotional experience. Both situations offer a brief sense of closeness and, of course, another goodbye. When you receive a sign, it can be helpful to take some space to process your experience in writing or out loud with a trusted person.

Depending on your cultural beliefs and upbringing, it may or may not feel realistic or appropriate to talk about this type of experience. Often, grieving people express some hesitation about sharing signs, as they fear being seen as silly—particularly if they were not engaged in spirituality prior to their loss. You may feel compelled to share an experience, but encounter loved ones who don't believe it. This could lead you to feel shame or to second-guess the sign. Try holding space for the disappointment that comes from not having your experience validated, and try to still honor it for yourself. Maintaining a connection often happens in small, quiet moments that are just for you. Some grievers ask their loved ones to send signs to show that they are still with them. Others do not, instead welcoming the signals if they happen to come through. When we want that communication so badly or hear others' sign stories but don't have our own, we might feel disappointment, frustration, loneliness, or skepticism about our own beliefs.

These feelings are entirely valid and can be tended to in many ways if a spiritual connection is important to us.

Reaching Out to the Great Unknown

We don't have to wait until we receive a sign to feel connected with our people. In fact, we can call our loved ones close to us in so many ways. Here are some of them.

Altar Building: Earlier, I shared that we can help ourselves through the waves of grief by creating an altar. Revisit chapter 5 for suggestions on what you may want to include on your altar and how you may opt to arrange it. Creating space for your person in your home may bolster a spiritual sense that they are present with you.

Visualization: You may also find connection through visualizing them when in a grounded state. For example, if you meditate, as you sit on the floor or meditation cushion, let your eyes close and try to call in a sense of your person as you breathe. Remove any pressure to clear your mind and instead focus on them. Can you feel any of their energy by picturing their face, their hands, their smile, their touch, their smell? Try not to worry about the details that don't surface and trust that whatever comes through is meant for the moment. You may also wish to try this when in *savasana*—a yoga pose in which you lie on the floor and relax. These practices may not only help us experience closeness but also soften emotional blockages, resulting in some release.

Talking to Them: Whether this is a desire sparked by events in your life (like good or bad news), a sign from them, or simply a moment of longing, you can speak to them. This is another area where many grieving folks fear judgment. In both individual and group therapy with the grieving, I have noticed that it can feel risky for people to admit that they do this, until I or others share that we maintain this practice also. You might find yourself talking to your person without having planned to. You might intentionally do this and it may even feel a little silly at first. When you speak out loud to them, notice how you feel before, during, and after. Pause to listen and notice what, if anything, comes through. If it's quiet, try not to panic or despair—this may not be the practice that works for you or it may not be the right moment to receive.

Letter Writing: This is another practice I describe in detail in chapter 5. If you feel uncomfortable speaking aloud or naturally tend to process via written word, this may be the most comforting conduit to your person. Feel free to write anything you would like to share with them— what is new in your world, where you are in your grief, questions you may have for them. The letter can be your channel for sending them these messages.

While it can be a source of comfort to reach your person in these ways, if it aligns with your beliefs, it is also not the only way to maintain a connection. Engaging spiritually with loved ones is not for everyone and it is not a requirement for integrating your grief.

Connecting Without Spiritual Beliefs

You can experience a sense of closeness to your loved one without believing that they are still existing in some form. All the activities I just described can be done and experienced as worthwhile without any belief in an afterlife. For you, connection may mean calling upon your person's memory. Nearly everything you can do to spiritually connect can also be done to remember, and feel gratitude for, the relationship you had with them. You can keep parts of the relationship alive for yourself by bringing their essence into your ongoing life, without needing to believe that their spirits are living within your atmosphere. For example, your altar—where you may display a photo of them and perhaps some trinkets related to them or your memories together—can simply honor that relationship and what it means to you. The altar can just be for you. If you engage in meditation or yoga, you can remember and visualize them during these practices, not necessarily to call their soul into the space, but for comfort. You can write a letter to them, releasing everything you need to say to experience catharsis, without needing to believe they will receive those words. You may even want to try speaking aloud to them. When you ask your person questions about a life decision like moving or a job, see if you can call in their voice and imagine how they would have responded. Even if you may not capture the exact words, see if you can feel the nature of it. Remember that you know them. Another way you may gain a sense of closeness is through taking up a hobby they enjoyed or connecting with a piece of art they loved—experiencing for yourself some of the life that they enjoyed. Much of connecting involves memory and if your memory feels shaky, this is understandable. There are ways to work with it.

Working with Memory

In some ways, memory can feel like all we have to grab onto after loss. So it becomes all the more precious and fragile. Before reading any further, pause to notice what you feel when this topic comes up. You might notice sadness or anxiety. Check in to see where your feelings are in the body and, if it feels supportive for you, give yourself the space to take a few deep breaths. Grief can bring up a very potent fear of forgetting—both specific memories and the general sense of what it felt like to be with our people.

The Fear of Forgetting

Years ago, I often feared that I would forget the sound of my mother's voice, her facial expressions, the way her palms felt against mine, or how she typically responded to something. I would find myself straining to produce some image, sound, or sentence, just to check that I still could. I would come up blank. Something happened in between trying to bring forth the memory and recognizing the blank emptiness that occurred afterward. It was anxiety. I was anxious about whether or not I still had the memories living inside of me. I would be struck with a preemptive fear of my inability to bring them to the surface. What would it mean if I was unable to recall the details of her? Maybe it would mean that I was left with nothing.

We often feel our memories are the last remnant of a person. Some keep the memories tucked away, theirs only to behold and shared with no one else. This is a place to practice discernment. Perhaps there are memories you wish to keep for yourself and there is something so special about that. Yet, there may be others you wish to share. Can you consider that sharing about your person does not mean giving them away? Maybe you could even bring some parts of them alive by speaking about them.

As frightening as it is to sit with a foggy memory, pushing and fighting our neural pathways to force memory hurts us more. We experience panic and freeze up, which might prevent us from accessing memories we truly do possess. There is another choice you can make. When you find yourself nervously wondering whether or not you remember, notice if you then feel a compulsion to try, and then see how it feels to let that urge pass. It may calm you to stop checking. If we relax our grip on the worry of not remembering, we might actually be free enough to do so. Allow memories to flow naturally, trusting that they will come when they come, and consider that maybe every detail isn't necessary and that remembering is more about the feeling. Think about people in your life who are living—do you remember the details of every instant you've spent with them? Probably not, but you do have a general sense of what you feel when you're with them. Perhaps you can reframe your relationship to memory so that this sense of them is what matters most. It's what we can hold onto and find our way back to when memories get lost in the shuffle of our ongoing lives.

One way to foster and build upon memories as they flow is to keep a memory log. This can be as simple as writing in a journal every time you receive a memory. Jot it down, letting it be whatever it is. It doesn't need to be flowery or totally coherent. Some of mine read this way: "In Dad's car, seeing my first sunshower" or "Hatboxes in Mum's closet." Sometimes those brief flashes of memory become seeds we can grow into more expansive memories and other times they will just remain seeds. Either way, they are still a portal to your person.

Being the Sole Keeper of Memories

A particularly sharp pang of grief can arise from the realization that you are the sole keeper of some memories. You might recall moments that you spent alone with someone who is no longer here—the one person who could remember those moments with you, but is unable to. You might notice that these memories can never be held by anyone else in quite the same way. This is a solemn truth to acknowledge, and you deserve adequate space to process it. You may feel lonely about possessing some memories on your own without them here to hold up the other end. You might even have difficulty trusting your own memory and believing it was all real, similar to having a fuzzy child-hood memory and wondering if it was actually a dream. You may find yourself looking or wishing for others to tell the story for you. But even if they were present and could fill in some gaps, the experience may have looked entirely different from their perspective.

So, where do all the past experiences go? They may either quietly live on within you and depart when you eventually do. Or they can be written on paper, spoken around a dinner table, maybe even carried down through the generations. There is no right or wrong choice—only the one that speaks to you. You might consider keeping some memories for yourself, taking a moment to be with them when they come up. You might share some with others, giving you and your person who died a chance to be witnessed. This is another way letter writing can be supportive, as you share the surfaced memory with your loved one who has died.

The Fear of Only Remembering the End

During a therapy session, James sits across from me and shares that when he remembers his late wife, he feels stuck on scenes of her aggressive illness. It was a time when he felt totally out of control and not emotionally resourced to handle the devastation that was occurring. While memories of her illness are not intruding on his day-to-day life as often, it is as though any prior memories—especially the happy ones—have been shoved aside to make way for the sharper images of her suffering. "I just hope the good memories come back," James says, simmering with tender vulnerability. James's wife died a little over eight months ago. After a lengthy process of settling affairs, he now has the space to begin processing his grief.

I validate his experience by saying, "You know, it's normal to find yourself stuck on those memories of the end right now." I explain what I'll share with you now: Trauma can have a significant impact on memory. Witnessing the end of a loved one's life or suddenly learning of it can be traumatic. This may make that point in time very blurry or, conversely, the traumatic images become imprinted in ways that take center stage in memory. Working with this is a matter of processing and surrendering. We may need to talk through the painful memories out loud, in order to make space for the happy ones. Just as we may need to surrender and trust that any memories will surface, we may need to similarly hold hope that over time we will be able to remember further back. When a memory crosses our mind, it won't always be sad. Maybe we will even smile or laugh out loud when we remember a funny moment.

Other Ways to Foster Memory

If you find that your connection feels acutely distant or it's challenging to remember the good times, there are some things you can do. Photos and videos can be a powerful tool for stimulating memory. Before you view them, check in with yourself about the timing and whether or not it is something you have the capacity to process. This may even be painful, at times. This practice of connecting puts us in touch with a beautiful kind of pain—beautiful because it is evidence of love, the stuff we come here for. You may want to do a grounding practice beforehand like mindful breathing, a body scan, or meditation in order to regulate your nervous system. This will help with the emotional activation of seeing and hearing them.

Another way we can try to stimulate memory and feel a sense of connection is by tapping into our olfactory sense. See if you happen to remember a product they used, for example, a perfume. Maybe you spot it in the background of a home video or find it mentioned in a text chain between the two of you. Even if it is not something you would otherwise use, consider buying a small bottle of it. Notice what comes up for you when you spray it. It may be a source of comfort that you could even add to an altar, if you have one. We can also experience a sense of closeness by going to a specific location, like their burial place, or somewhere you spent time with them. While being there might make the loss feel more alive and raw, it may also enliven your memories and your ongoing connection. Though we may experience challenges remaining connected to our people, it is very possible to do so when we have the capacity to trust, hope, and creatively expand our notion of what connection can be.

Sustaining Love and Unfinished Business

Staying connected to our people is not just about feeling their presence or holding our memories close. When we stay connected, we may find that these relationships continue to help us and evolve as we do. For some of us, the person who had to leave is also the one who gifted us with a love so sustaining that it allows us to be without them and, alongside the grief, live fully. If we tap into the feeling of their love for us, we can place our focus there, experiencing gratitude for ever having had them. If it speaks to you, a phrase you can return to is: *The love they gave me lives on just like the love I have for them.* When the relationship was largely positive and we know we were loved by them, it's as if they leave us with most of what we need. However, we also lose loved ones with whom we had deeply complicated relationships. Grief for them involves further tasks.

Grief develops extra layers when it wraps around a relationship that was complex. When you lose them, you also lose the opportunity for addressing things unsaid, for making amends. They are not here to work it out with us. For example, maybe there was a great harm done, by them or by you, and it was never truly discussed or thoroughly processed. Perhaps you find yourself reflecting on this harm and wishing you could bring your reflections, new and old, to them. Part of your grief integration and maintaining a relationship with them from beyond may involve working through what happened and repairing a rupture on your own. Grief therapy can be a powerful tool for this kind of processing that helps us to uncover elements of our relationship and maybe even release what we no longer wish to carry. Even if your relationship with your loved one was largely positive, you might find that in therapy, you uncover a habit, part of your personality, or a self-limiting belief that appears tied to them. This is a natural part of reviewing our life story through loss and, in fact, the pull to process these realizations is almost proof that relationships go on despite death.

Guilt can be a pesky companion and it might rear its head again, especially if you were raised to not speak ill of the dead. However, acknowledging that your person and your relationship with them were complex is okay. Often you're just recalling the truth, and that doesn't have to mean you love them any less. Choosing to stay connected means staying open to it all—not just the good stuff but also the hard times. Grief accompanies both.

As I sifted through some home movies, I once came across my mother filming the closure of my father's video store a few months after his death. In the movie, she asks me to narrate and I'm upbeat as I guide her through the store. It's sad to watch because it was the lowest point of our family's life thus far. Yet, I'm glad and even grateful that I have footage of this place because I can smell the interior like I was just there.

You don't have to keep all these thoughts about the relationship locked up inside. Perhaps in your letter to your loved one, this is what you write about, sharing with them all that you have discovered and all that you need them to hear. If you are drawn to visualization, give yourself some time in a quiet, private space to imagine you are sitting with your person. Envision yourself speaking to them (or you may speak aloud) about the hard parts of your dynamic, what you have learned, what you wish to have validated. Visualize them calmly engaging and listening, even if this isn't how it would have unfolded in the past. You might even imagine words of affirmation. If this feels intimidating to do alone, consider asking your therapist if they can assist you in an empty chair exercise, so you can speak with your person and have support processing this. Engaging in one of these practices may be what you need in order to continue on, alongside your grief.

Letting Them Live Through Us

Yes, we may fear that if we lose memories, we will have nothing left. While a daunting prospect, this wouldn't be true even if it were to happen. Why? Because our people are part of us. You are marked by your connection with them, changed not just by their absence but impacted by the presence they had in your life. Sometimes, staying close to this truth is aided by letting them live through us. Consider the following invitations to do so.

Share Them with Others: There are days when we may need to reflect on their deaths and voice what losing them has done to us. On other days, when we have the capacity, we may be empowered by sharing stories about their life with others. My mother had a lot of pain in her life, but a lot of joy too. When I think of her, I don't just think of her sickness, I think of her sense of humor, her ability to laugh at herself, her beauty, her style, her quiet wisdom and confidence, her gracefulness. I want her to exist out in the world as all that she was, not just how she slipped away from this world. This takes time.

Embody Them: If you feel comfortable tapping into some memory, read on. If you don't, feel free to pause and return to this page later. Think back to one of the traits you most closely associate with your person—perhaps it's their generosity, their honesty, or their optimism. Whatever trait it may be, set an intention to embody it out in the world this week. Notice how it makes you feel, for example, to do an act of kindness that they would have done. Alternatively, think back to an activity you associate with them, perhaps one you often did together. It doesn't have to be anything exciting, for example, I feel close to my father when I do weekend errands. Do that thing and see if you can feel them there.

Keep Their Belongings Alive: If you have belongings of theirs, consider self-adorning with them or displaying them in your home. It may seem like a small, simple act—and it is. Take care to not underestimate the power of subtly keeping their memory around you. When we put on their jewelry or an item of their clothing, we are keeping them just a little closer. For decorating with their presence in mind, allow yourself to think outside the box. Frame a card or short note they wrote to you and hang it somewhere you'll see often.

Live on Their Behalf: We can also mindfully live a little on their behalf. Think about something they wanted to do, from traveling to reading a particular book, going to a certain music concert or a specific sports event. Ask yourself if this is something you would like to do as well. If it feels aligned, consider doing that activity. Try to be discerning and realistic, so as not to place pressure on yourself. You don't have to climb Mount Everest for them if that is far from being your thing. You are simply considering ways to honor them and what they loved and longed for.

Final Thoughts

Over time, as we integrate our grief and feel less consistently weighed down by it, we free up space inside of us to stay connected. It's vital to remember that the connection is always there for us to tap into. When we feel disconnected, we can seek out ways to return to them through whatever brings us closer in our unique bond. This helps us realize what is always there, over and over. We can do this, and should feel free to, regardless of our spiritual beliefs. We may even heal the fractures in the relationship with our person, in our own way, on our own time. Our connections are dynamic and unsevered by death, though it is natural to fear losing them. May we remember that while the details of our memories can blur at times, there is no true forgetting.

Early on, it may feel like grief is what tethers us to our people. But in truth, it's not all we get to keep. It can be terrifying to contemplate that the depth of our pain will ease, and the loss will remain. We might even feel it is almost a service to our people to remain bound to our mourning, as the concept of joy becomes a betrayal. Trust that you do not need to cling to that early darkness in order to stay connected. To slowly, softly move in the direction of joy is to move in the direction of the person you lost. Trust that finding happiness again will not take you further away from them, instead it will bring you closer. That first big laugh, that first sigh of relief, that first genuine smile. That is where they are too.

REFLECTION QUESTION

When and where do you feel closest to the person you lost?

CHAPTER 10

Lighting the Path

Wherever you are in your process, imagine that you are further down the path of this life shaped, in part, by grief. The murky darkness that once felt endless and consuming may feel far away now. You may only vaguely remember the sensation of being in grief's depths, where you believed you would never feel like "you" again, where you believed Earth would always feel like an uninhabitable planet without your person. You are integrating your grief, letting it weave its way in and out of your life, tending to the swells of emotion as they come. You are quieting the outside noise that encourages you to ignore it—and this has paid off. As a result, you have freed up some internal space to experience contentment, even joy. This process will be ongoing, but you may feel more resourced to meet it.

When we come to this place where grief and joy coexist as they take turns stepping to the forefront, and we can accept ourselves through it all, we have an opportunity. We can look back and notice others starting out on the path, and we can light some of the way for their journey. When able, we can lovingly companion others who grieve, even if on a small scale. Early on in grief, they need to see that somebody else made it through. When they see someone who survived and is maybe even strengthened by the ordeal of early grief, they gain hope. Hope is important. We can hold ourselves up as living proof that, *No, it won't feel this way forever,* while also honoring their unique experience and timing. All we have to do to begin is check in on our willingness. When presented with this of idea of lighting the way for others, what comes up for you? What does the voice inside say? Is it dismissive? You may ask, *What would I have to share?* If it sounds pressured, you might say, *That sounds daunting. What if I say or do the wrong thing?* You may feel annoyed and insist, *I still have my own stuff to be with. Why would I take on anyone else's pain?* You could also feel hopeful and wonder, *Maybe I can give someone else the support I didn't have.* Keep this in mind as you read the next section.

Willingness and Capacity

The willingness of others to talk about what really happens in grief is what helps us feel less alone and alienated by the world around us. Despite loss and grief happening to every person at some point in their life, these events are often shrouded in silence—except for the voices of those who feel compelled to share. They may share directly or from a distance as we read about their grief or watch their film on the subject. Everyone needs someone they can connect with in this experience. When we lose someone, we may develop a tender sense that everything can be lost. When others are in this, prodding their way through darkness, we can be there to remind them that while many things can be lost, not everything will be.

Take a moment to consider if anyone threw you a lifeline. Maybe someone reached out to let you know that they were there for you because they could, on some level, connect to what you were going through. What was helpful about this? It may have even been as simple as someone conveying, *Hey, I see you.* If no one comes to mind, I'm very sorry you went through this alone. Instead, remember what you needed in a support person but didn't receive.

Grievers need people in their lives who won't look away and who instead recognize grief won't ever be over, though the way it shows up may change. We need people who are not thinking about the timeline. They show interest in attuning to where we are and being there with us. Now, the people who may have showed up for you didn't have to do this, just as you don't either. I want to be clear that you are under no obligation to be of service to others who are grieving or to share your story in doing so.

Boundaries

You may feel protective of your loss story and of your energy. After all, you have worked so hard to conserve it. This is okay. Think again of that person who may have supported you. Maybe they related and told you about their experience. Maybe they simply listened to you when you needed to talk. Maybe they helped you find some distraction when you needed to suspend reality and temporarily get away from it all. Do you think that they shared *everything* about their journey? They may have shared what they felt would be helpful, but they may not have dished out every detail. It's likely they haven't discovered everything there is to discover about their own grief yet, even if it began many years ago, because grief is ongoing. It's not necessary to share it all in order to be supportive. In fact, we even want to be cautious about centering sharing in our support efforts, as it can shift the spotlight away from the person you're helping when they really need the focus to be on them and their raw pain. Was your support person available at all hours? Hopefully, for both of your sakes, they showed up when they truly felt able to. In addition to checking in with your capacity to support other grievers, it will be important for you to cultivate a keen sense of your own boundaries. It is a word we hear often and it may even begin to lose its meaning as this happens, sort of like those platitudes.

Boundaries are essentially our protective guardrails for what we are willing to do and allow ourselves to participate in. We create boundaries for ourselves in order to maintain our emotional (or even physical) safety. They help foster genuine connections that are not rife with resentment. Boundaries are helpful, not harmful, because they help us focus on wisely choosing our own actions rather than controlling another. For example, if you are in relationship with someone who is relying on excessive alcohol consumption to cope with life's challenges, whether or not you encourage them to seek support, you may set a boundary with them around it. Rather than saying, "You are not allowed to drink," which would be an attempt to control, you can say "I am not going to be around you while you drink." This focuses on what you will or will not do.

The more we practice setting and holding boundaries throughout various facets of our lives, the more natural it becomes. Sometimes, people find it challenging to set boundaries for fear of upsetting the other person. While others may not make you feel *good* about your boundary, their ability to respect it may be a strong sign of the integrity of the relationship. Boundaries benefit you and also your relationships because when we agree to things that do not sit right with us, we can develop resentment toward people we care about.

We can create boundaries around our grief support efforts as well. These boundaries may be related to the specific ways we give support, the timing of it, the content we share, and how all this shifts depending on the closeness of the relationship. Take a moment to consider the following questions, to begin forming some guidelines for yourself.

In what ways might I feel able to support someone who is grieving? There are many ways to give of yourself when someone you care about is going through life-altering loss. In chapter 3, we checked in with what you needed when in survival mode and how others could step in. Your own support could be quality time when you bear witness, whether the grief is discussed or not. It could mean cooking or cleaning or running errands for someone. Notice what feels aligned with your capacity and how that intersects with what they need—this is how you can be of great service.

What parts of my story do I feel reasonably comfortable to share with someone who is grieving? Grieving people may want to hear if the devastating and bizarre things they're noticing are "normal" and they may want to hear how you got through it all. Bear in mind that we are not controlling (we simply can't control another person) what they ask or how they respond. We are sharing only what we feel freely comfortable to answer. For example, say someone asks about details of your loved one's illness and discussing that lies outside of your boundaries. Rather than saying, "Don't ask me something like that," you can say something like, "That's a part I'm not up for sharing or getting into right now." Consider the nuanced difference between privacy and secrecy. You may wish to keep your story, or parts of it, private. This is distinct from keeping it secret. Privacy may mean discernment and sharing with some people, though not all. Secrecy may mean sharing with almost no one. Privacy says *this is sacred*, while secrecy says *this is shameful*. If reading the latter sends a twinge of resonance through you, shame may be something to investigate in your therapy.

Are there parts of my story I only feel comfortable to share with others who are very close to me? What are they? It is reasonable and realistic to notice that some of our relationships are closer and deeper than others. Note that sharing more vulnerability is a sure way to deepen a relationship, if this is something we want. The choice may come down to how long you've known the person seeking your help and how much history you share as you lived through hard times together. But it may also come down to the feeling you experience being with them. It's likely you'll feel more inclined to share more with people who in the past have actively listened, asked before giving advice, and accepted you without trying to change you or your feelings.

How do I know if it is or is not the right time for me to help or share? Capacity is vital to consider when supporting someone. If we are deep in our stuff, we may not have as much room to welcome another person's grief. Keep in mind that boundaries can also serve as a sort of forcefield that keeps our emotions distinct from another person's emotions. This isn't being cold—it's taking care to not absorb their emotions as your own, keeping what's theirs and yours separate enough that you can actually bear witness. Then you can extend care without being pulled under, into a state that drains you and leaves you unable to help. Before stepping into a grief support role, take some time to check in with your capacity, how full your cup is or isn't, and decide from there if and how much you can give without depleting yourself. We can't pour from empty cups and we all deserve to experience the feeling of fullness.

You also do not need to form some grand commitment to always be open about your grief. You may move through seasons when you feel the need to go dark, to be quiet and in solitude with your grief, no matter how much time has passed. You can move fluidly from not sharing to sharing and back again, because you may have varying needs at different points in time. The important thing is that you communicate about these changes with people in your life, especially those who may come to you for support. It is never too late to change the way you interact with others and the world around your grief. You can always start sharing your grief, even if for years you didn't feel ready. Or you can focus on processing on your own after previously being very open.

When making disclosures that you live with grief, you may have to likewise experiment, just as you did when you were first venturing out into the world after loss. Continue to find what feels right for you as you go along. If you find yourself doing and saying things out of social pressure and later regretting it, you may strongly benefit from setting clear boundaries for yourself and writing down the answers to these questions. If you tend to move intuitively through life and find that this feels supportive for you, it may not feel aligned to create several detailed guidelines. Instead, give yourself some room right now to reflect on this.

Connecting with Fellow Grievers

When we walk along our healing path, we may become unrecognizable to those who felt they knew us as we grieved in silence. Others may deeply embrace us and want to bear witness to the depth of who we are. As we considered in chapter 6, this is a big reason why relationships change in grief. The death of someone instrumental in our lives can set us on a path to seek out new experiences, create more life for ourselves, and discover more about this new version of us. Who we become will likely not be for everyone. Loss and grief can change the direction of our lives, softening and opening us to pain we've never known before. They also bring us to new people we connect with, and care about, deeply. If you feel enlivened by this idea and compelled to shine a light for others, let's explore some practical ways you can do this.

How Can We Light the Path for Others?

Most simply, and sometimes most meaningfully, we can provide some light in the dark for other grievers by simply reaching out. Has anyone in your world experienced a big loss since you did? Did you reach out to them? If you didn't, was there a part of you that wanted to? If it was a matter of capacity, consider how you gauged this for yourself. These are things to keep in mind if a future instance arises, as it is likely to, given that we all experience loss. If it feels right for you, and you have the capacity and space in your life, consider reaching out with an offer to connect. For example, you might say, "I just want you to know that I'm thinking of you. I don't know your experience exactly because we're all unique, but I know that this is the hardest thing to go through. I just want you to know that the door is open if you ever need space to talk, and I mean it."

If appropriate given the level of connection you have with this person, consider doing a tangible act of care. As you extend support, see if you can simultaneously hold your knowledge of what felt helpful for you with the knowledge that what every individual needs in grief will differ. This is wisdom coupled with humility. The channel of connection may also run the other way. If you are open about your grief in your family, friend groups, communities, or even online spaces, you may end up having people in the early depths of grief reach out to you. I have had the honor of being contacted by people with varying levels of connection. We have met each other in the sacredness of being on this side of life in ways I never expected.

If this openness appeals to you or sparks some curiosity, take time to consider your interests and skills to see how you can channel them. Do you like to write? Maybe start a blog or attend a writing workshop. Do you like to organize? Perhaps brainstorm an event. If you are an artist and grief is surfacing in your work, consider sharing it. If you feel called to be of service, consider looking into *death doula* training that can prepare you to support the dying as well as their families. If you do, find a training that takes place in-person or offers a group-study format, so you can form a network with others who deeply honor grief. If you work with children or adolescents, you may also wish to volunteer at a grief camp. The possibilities are endless if you are open to thinking creatively about what you have to offer and how you feel most called to help.

How This Helps Us

Something else you might consider doing, particularly if you want to continue reflecting along your own path, is joining a grief support group. Though you might feel shame come up around the idea of getting support for a loss that happened years ago, it is actually never too late. When I offer grief groups, I do not place a time restriction on when the loss occurred. Everyone deserves to give their grief room to breathe, to let it come out into the open, in all its iterations over time. Grief doesn't respect our timelines, as people may not grieve until years after a death when they finally break through survival mode. Not everyone has the support and the tools to dive right in. Often deep exploration early after loss is unrealistic. Our psyches and emotions first need time to acclimate to the reality of it. Your experience in group may be twofold: You can explore your own continued grief aloud and you can be a voice of wisdom for others who are in the early part of their process. All vantage points and unique perspectives are worthy. This variation makes for a rich group dynamic.

Grief has changed us. It is like swapping out a pair of glasses for a new prescription that makes us see the world differently. Loss can create a life overhaul and spark reflections that guide us to desire new connections. We may even realize that some relationships were tied to parts of ourselves we are ready to outgrow. Within us, grief does reveal new needs and interests, clarified values, and more simply a yearning for a temperature check that says, *Yes, I am not the only one who feels this way.* There is a gentle ease that comes with knowing grief and being around others who know grief too. There's a sense of understanding the unspoken through a connection that makes explaining, in some instances, almost unnecessary. We may find that other grievers understand the many faces of grief, invisible to the untrained eye. They know that it does not only look like being down on your knees, uncontrollably wailing. They know how it surfaces in quiet moments, silent acknowledgments, flittering realizations of absence. Grief can feel utterly singular, and at the same time, bring us together in ways we can't envision beforehand.

Given that we exist within a dominant culture that isn't equipped to support us, grieving people find and connect with each other in order to heal, whether through therapy groups events or within a larger social group. This sounds like people saying: "No, you're not crazy." "Yes, people really do say those things." "Yes, it really is wrong and so hurtful." "I know, I can't believe this is forever either." "We're going to make it, somehow." Some people on the outside of grief come across as though they fear contracting our sadness, as though it's contagious. They sympathize, perhaps, but don't empathize because that would mean imagining life-altering loss for themselves. Instead, they consciously or unconsciously distance themselves from our grief. It is too frightening to consider the truth that one day, they too will be in our shoes—such is the risk we take in loving anyone. We need spaces where no one is worried about "catching" our grief because they have theirs. They are in on the big secret truth that this is part of life—a significant part. Finding other grievers to connect with helps us protect our other relationships with those who have not experienced grief yet, because when we have our needs met, we feel less resentment. We can, maybe, accept those other friends and loved ones for who they are, what they can give us, and what they can't because they just haven't lived it yet.

When we hold each other up, it can be enlightening. We're not only lamenting, although we, of course, need that too. Our connections can be active and thought-provoking, energizing even. When we let ourselves be mirrors to one another, we reflect and uncover new layers. There is always more we can learn about what our losses mean to us and what they mean for our lives, if we want to seek that out. Sharing stories of what we have been through, and being witnessed by others who "get it," isn't a one-way street of support. It helps us too, in ways that we never have to be above receiving. It can even be empowering when we reflect on what we've found in grief. Until we have a conversation with someone else, we may not be able to step outside of ourselves for a moment and say, *Wow, I can't believe that I can do this, that I have this knowledge to give, that I actually survived.*

Sure, talking about grief with each other isn't fascinating and beautiful all of the time. It's also about letting the darkness come into the light. We might be able to make the morbid jokes only we feel comfortable with together. We can name what is unfixable and just be there together in that without fear of someone chiming in to offer a way out that doesn't actually exist. When we gather, there are so many ways we participate in others' healing, beyond the healing of those in the room.

Maybe you've noticed the tight-lipped smile you give when a new acquaintance assumes your loved one is still alive and you contemplate how you will correct them. Ideally, people would not make assumptions about what our families look like and who we do or do not have in our lives. Hopefully, following such an interaction with you, that person will give this some consideration. Creating more openness about grief increases grief awareness, which doesn't just benefit those of us who have known deep loss. It also benefits those who will one day join us in this knowing. Grief awareness is for everyone. It is a necessary culture shift only waiting for us to create it.

Helping People Who Couldn't Help Us

Sometimes, when we're further along the path, we may be summoned to support a grieving person who had little to no knowledge or experience at the time that *we* needed support. They may have been one of those people who just didn't *get it* when we really needed someone to understand. Hopefully, you found that person in someone else. Still, their inability to help may have created distance or even a rupture in your relationship, even if they were well-intentioned but inadvertently harmful. Maybe they said something insensitive, maybe they didn't acknowledge your grief or check in on how you were doing. If an instance like this occurs, notice what comes up for you when you learn their news. You might feel less willing to reach out if the anger or resentment remains present and the relationship has become distant. You may also feel compelled to check in on them. While loss can create distance, it also has a way of cutting right through the conflicts we once felt fired up about. Is there an opportunity for repair here? There is no right or wrong. This is simply another place to check in with yourself. At this time, what feels important to you, what do you feel able to do without bringing harm to yourself, and what actions feel most aligned with your values?

Connecting with other people who carry grief and lending a hand to those still learning how to exist in this complex reality is a worthwhile and important effort. It is part of how we continue to process and grow alongside our losses. When we reach out in a way that aligns with our capacity and boundaries, we fill our own cup and the cup of the person before us. We contribute to a shift toward greater openness about what loss is really like and more adept responsiveness to the realities of grief. Why should something so fundamental, so guaranteed, be concealed by shame? Every one of us, touched by grief, can be part of this great uncovering so that no one ever has to be so alone.

No Pressure to Be the Expert

You may have heard of a *wounded healer* before. Swiss psychiatrist and psychologist Carl Jung coined this concept, originally termed the "wounded physician" in the context of psychotherapy. Jung believed that it is the physician's wound that actually enables them to heal someone else, just to the extent that they have been able to heal for themselves (2024). Essentially, the hard things you have been through may be exactly what allow you to help someone else through hard things. By drawing from your own wounds to be with those of another, you bring forth your personal wisdom, your open heart, your willingness. These are gifts and putting them into action offers a sense of purpose.

You don't have to believe you are an expert in order to have something to offer. Just as we ask of those who have not yet experienced grief, try to focus less on saying or doing the wrong thing and more on attuning to *what is* for the grieving person in front of you. You can't know what their path forward will look like exactly because, the truth is, you don't know what the future will look like for you either. What we do know is that loss disregards the plans we had and also, somehow, creates new possibilities for us if we are willing to seek them out. Own your knowledge and also take care not to place pressure on yourself to gain ultimate mastery. Growing through grief doesn't mean winning a battle with it, outsmarting it, stamping it out. It's about learning how to be with it and continue welcoming the changes it brings. Seeing this modeled in someone else is impactful enough. And when they're ready, we can even share that as horrible as loss is, as much as it cuts us open, that opening is where we let more love in, more appreciation for the little things, and of course, for life itself.

REFLECTION QUESTION

How and why do you personally light the path forward for the grieving people in your world?

CONCLUSION

This is a difficult book for me to end. There are infinite threads we could pull at and I would like to just stay here with you. But I imagine, gladly, that you have some things to get on to in life. I'll leave you with a few thoughts. Grief is forever—and that's not the bad news it sounds like. It is an endless well of wisdom, formed by a deep bond. What you can draw from it will give you the keys to every locked door you come across in life, helping you open them, strengthening you to get through them all. Grief totally breaks us down and also makes us appreciate sunrises and laughter and the person who holds the door when you're having a terrible morning. Then grief turns you into the person who holds the door.

Growing through grief is not all doom and gloom. Loss isn't going to be the only thing you can feel or what paints the broad strokes of your daily life, even if you're in the depths right now. In fact, I hope you will find that as you integrate your grief, you feel stronger for it. By actively meeting grief when it comes up, we release some of the pressure and it becomes something we fear less and less. We develop deeper self-knowing than we may have otherwise possessed, riding our waves of emotion, feeling confident in our ability to weather the most difficult storms. We are not merely setting out to avoid further pain or to avoid becoming hardened into bitterness. We don't have to do this work from a place of fear, thinking, *If I don't face it, it's going to sneak up and hurt me.* Instead we do this work from a place of ground-edness within, even if the actual ground beneath sometimes feels shaky. People who live with immense grief are some of the most admirable amongst us. We walk a little differently—empowered by the very tenderness we carry.

It is also safe to loosen your grip on the pain. Your relationship with your beloved person is never going to go away or be less important because you do that. I have journeyed on the path to suppressing my pain and it took me further away from those I've lost. I decided to change this, just as you are. When I journeyed even further into the reintegration of that pain, I returned to myself, though changed in some ways, and I returned to the loved ones I grieve. This only continues. I look forward to the process for myself, and for you. Keep surrendering to the changes and know that you can revisit parts of this book over time, as needed. You are not meant finish it at any particular point in your grief, just as you were not meant to start it at any particular point other than when felt right for you. The more you integrate, the more space within you will free up to remember the good in a way that makes you smile, helps you share about them, and keeps them a part of this world. Grief doesn't shrink into nothingness. It remains because it is love sustained and we grow through it.

It is often easier to see growth in others than to see our own, easier to observe how they have transformed than witness that transformation in ourselves. Take a moment to notice where you've been and where you are now, maybe even where you might be going, and whether or not it feels okay to not know. (It is okay.) Remember something that I see in you: People who live in honor of someone they love carry a special light. If you choose to shine that onto others, you are only continuing to honor your person. How special to find light in the dark, to turn on the switch and help someone else see that there is a way through. Loss enhances our tenderness and this, though painful, is a good thing—a beautiful thing. We are that much more alive for it. And we know how precious that is.

ACKNOWLEDGMENTS

My parents, Karen and Billy Zappala, are the heart of this book. I thank them for loving me, others, and each other well, for living with joy and dying with grace.

This book could not have been written were it not for my husband, Riyad Mammadyarov. Thank you for your unwavering support, belief, and partnership.

I would not be doing this work, much less standing if not for my sister, Brittany Acciavatti. I give you my deepest gratitude. Your unmatched selflessness and sisterhood made my healing possible, and by extension, the healing of so many others. You deserve all of the good you've given tenfold. I would choose us and do this all again, every time.

A very special thank you to Tom Acciavatti for doing the extraordinary.

To Vivi Acciavatti, Billy Acciavatti, and Fiona Acciavatti, thank you for enlivening my curiosity, creativity, and sense of play. Should you ever need them, I hope these words can hold you. I will too.

To the village that sustained me as I grew up with grief: Anne Russell, Joni Marks, Peter Marks, Terri Webber, Meredith Marks, Jonathan Marks, Ashley Marks, Kevin Russell, Matthew Russell, Shannon Kjellsen, Gillian Galen, Michael Moresco, Robert Cleary.

To Kamilla Sardarova and Elmar Mammadyarov for your love and encouragement.

To Lisa Zappala and Susan Zappala for helping me keep memories alive.

To Dominique Troy and Gina Moffa for being with me since the start of this journey.

To Alua Arthur for the end-of-life education I have been fortunate enough to receive.

To Jennye Garibaldi for championing this tender work and providing me an opportunity I will never take for granted. To Madison Davis and Elizabeth Hollis Hansen for your support in the creation of this work.

To the incredible therapists and mentors who have supported and shaped me as a clinician: Laurie Godfrey, Alana Barlia, Sienna Chu, Alana Carvalho, Lindsey Pratt, Elizabeth Merrick, Teresa Hurst, Lynn Kaplan.

REFERENCES

American Psychiatric Association. 2013. *Diagnostic and statistical manual of mental disorders* (5th ed.). https://doi.org/10.1176/appi. books.9780890425596

American Psychological Association. 2018, April 19. APA dictionary of psychology. https://dictionary.apa.org/dissociation

Aron, A., Aron, E.N., & Smollan, D. 1992. Inclusion of other in the self scale and the structure of interpersonal closeness. *Journal of Personality and Social Psychology, 63*, 596–612. https://doi. org/10.1037/0022-3514.63.4.596

Boelen, P.A. 2017. Self-identity after bereavement: Reduced self-clarity and loss-centrality in emotional problems after the death of a loved one. *The Journal of Nervous and Mental Disease, 205*(5), 405–408. https://psycnet.apa.org/doi/10.1097/NMD.0000000000000660

Calhoun, L. G., Tedeschi, R. G., Cann, A., and Hanks, E.A. 2010. Positive outcomes following bereavement: Paths to posttraumatic growth. *Psychologica Belgica, 50*(1-2), 125–143. https://doi.org/10.5334/pb-50-1-2-125

Den Elzen, K. 2021. Therapeutic writing through the lens of the grief memoir and dialogical self theory. *Journal of Constructivist Psychology, 34*(2), 218–230. https://doi.org/10.1080/10720537.2020.1717136

Didion, J. 2005. *The Year of Magical Thinking.* New York, NY: Knopf.

Eisma, M. C., de Lang, T. A., Boelen, P. A. 2020. How thinking hurts: Rumination, worry, and avoidance processes in adjustment to bereavement. *Clinical Psychology & Psychotherapy, 27*(4), 548–558. https://doi.org/10.1002/cpp.2440

Emanuel, E. J. and Emanuel, L. L. 1998. The promise of a good death. *The Lancet, 351*, SII21–SII29. https://doi.org/10.1016S0140-6736(98)90329-4

Fagundes, C. P., Brown, R. L., Chen, M. A., Murdock, K. W., Saucedo, L., LeRoy, A., Wu, E. L., Garcini, L. M., Shahane, A. D., Baameur, F., Heijnen, C. 2019. Grief, depressive symptoms, and inflammation in the spousally bereaved. *Psychoneuroendocrinology, 100*, 190–197. https://doi.org/10.1016j.psyneuen.2018.10.006

Fleming, V., dir. *The Wizard of Oz*. 1939; Culver City, CA: Metro-Goldwyn-Mayer. Max.

Harris, C. B., Brookman, R., & O'Connor, M. 2023. It's not who you lose, it's who you are: Identity and symptom trajectory in prolonged grief. *Current Psychology, 42*, 11223–11233. https://doi.org/10.1007/s12144-021-02343-w

Jackson, L.L. 2015. *The Light Between Us: Stories from Heaven. Lessons for the Living*. New York, NY: Penguin Random House.

Jung, C. G. 2024. *Collected Works of C. G. Jung, Vol 16: Practice of Psychotherapy*, edited by Gerhard Adler and R. F.C. Hull. Princeton, NJ: Princeton University Press.

Konkolÿ Thege, B., Pilling, J., Cserháti, Z., and Kopp, M.S. 2012. Mediators between bereavement and som üatic symptoms. *BMC Family Practice, 13*, 59. https://doi.org/10.1186/1471-2296-13-59

Kübler-Ross, E. 1975. *Death: The Final Stage of Growth*. New Jersey: Prentice-Hall.

Linehan, M. 2015. *DBT® Skills Training Manual* (2nd ed.). New York, NY: Guilford Press.

O'Connor, M. F. 2022. *The Grieving Brain*. New York, NY: HarperOne.

Rogers, C. 1975. Empathic: An unappreciated way of being. *The Counseling Psychologist, 5*(2), 2–10. https://doi.org/10.1177/001100007500500202

Stanley, B. and Brown, G. K. 2012. Safety planning intervention: A brief intervention to mitigate suicide risk. *Cognitive and Behavioral Practice* 19(2): 256–264.

Stroebe, M. and Schut, H. 1999. The dual process model of coping with bereavement: Rationale and description. *Death Studies, 23(3)*, 197–224. https://doi.org/10.1080/074811899201046

Thomsen, D. K., Lundorff, M., Damkier, A., and O'Connor, M. 2018. Narrative identity and grief reactions: A prospective study of bereaved partners. *Journal of Applied Research in Memory and Cognition, 7*(3), 412–421. https://doi.org/10.1016/j.jarmac.2018.03.011

Toller, P. W. 2008. Bereaved parents' negotiation of identity following the death of a child. *Communication Studies, 59*(4), 306–321. https://doi.org/10.1080/10510970802467379

U.S. Department of labor. "Funeral Leave." Accessed April 28, 2024. https://www.dol.gov/general/topic/benefits-leave/funeral-leave.

Wehrman, E. C. 2023. "I don't even know who I am": Identity reconstruction after the loss of a spouse. *Journal of Social and Personal Relationships 2023, 40*(4) 1250–1276. https://doi.org/10.1177/02654075221127399

Alex Mammadyarov, LMHC, is a New York-based psychotherapist and writer forging new standards for the ways we grapple with grief. She works individually with people who are processing all types of grief, including the loss of loved ones to both death and estrangement, as well as those going through transitions, encountering challenges in their interpersonal relationships, experiencing anxiety, working through trauma, codependency, or seeking to develop a stronger relationship with themselves. Alex holds a dual master's degree in counseling psychology and mental health counseling from Teachers College, Columbia University. Additionally, Alex has obtained training as a death doula from Alua Arthur's Going with Grace End of Life Training Program, and offers group therapy for those looking to process grief from the loss of a parent.

Alex has been a guest on numerous podcasts, and she's been interviewed on the subject of grief by *Psychology Today* and Keys Soulcare (a wellness brand founded by Alicia Keys). Alex has been a guest blogger on *Remembering a Life*, and she's also been featured in articles on *Pop Sugar* and *Sunday Riley*. Her popular Instagram account is a combination of compassionate, affirming notes on healing and honest conversations for those dealing with death and living with loss.

Foreword writer **Marisa Renee Lee** is an award-winning author, advocate, entrepreneur, and leading voice in navigating grief and uncertainty. As CEO of Beacon Advisors and founder of the Grief is Love Research Project, she's committed to helping people thrive during challenging times. She is author of *Grief is Love: Living with Loss*.

MORE BOOKS from
NEW HARBINGER PUBLICATIONS

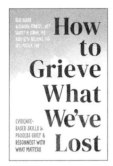
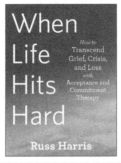
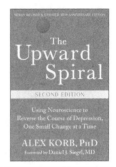
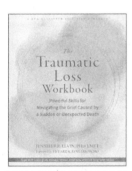
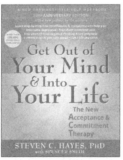
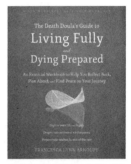

Did you know there are **free tools** you can download for this book?

Free tools are things like **worksheets, guided meditation exercises**, and **more** that will help you get the most out of your book.

You can download free tools for this book—whether you bought or borrowed it, in any format, from any source—from the New Harbinger website. All you need is a NewHarbinger.com account. Just use the URL provided in this book to view the free tools that are available for it. Then, click on the "download" button for the free tool you want, and follow the prompts that appear to log in to your NewHarbinger.com account and download the material.

You can also save the free tools for this book to your **Free Tools Library** so you can access them again anytime, just by logging in to your account! Just look for this button on the book's free tools page.

+ Save this to my free tools library